The MIDWIFE'S Pregnancy and Childbirth BOOK

The MIDWIFE'S Pregnancy and Childbirth BOOK

Having Your Baby Your Way

MARION McCARTNEY, CNM
ANTONIA VAN DER MEER

HENRY HOLT AND COMPANY
New York

LIBRARY OF CONGRESS CATALOGING-IN-PUBLICATION DATA
McCartney, Marion.
The midwife's pregnancy and childbirth book : having your baby
your way / Marion McCartney and Antonia van der Meer.—1st ed.
p. cm.
ISBN 0-8050-1049-1
1. Pregnancy. 2. Childbirth. I. Van der Meer, Antonia.
II. Title.
RG525.M384 1990
618.2'4—dc20   89-39853
                                                         CIP

Henry Holt books are available at special discounts for bulk pur-
chases for sales promotions, premiums, fund-raising, or educational
use. Special editions or book excerpts can also be created to
specification.

For details contact:
Special Sales Director
Henry Holt and Company, Inc.
115 West 18th Street
New York, New York 10011

First Edition

Designed by Kathryn Parise
Printed in the United States of America
Recognizing the importance of preserving the written word, Henry
Holt and Company, Inc., by policy, prints all of its first editions on
acid-free paper.∞

1   3   5   7   9   10   8   6   4   2

Photographs courtesy of Fred Ward

NOTE: This book is designed to guide and educate on the choices
available for childbirth. From time to time the authors recommend
that you consult your physician in a variety of situations. So, while
we hope our book will help you in making your decision, it should
not be used as a substitute for medical advice.

This book is dedicated to James Duncan Brew, Jr., my teacher, physician, and friend.

Thanks to Jan, Barbara, Mary, Carlene, and Cindy, who covered my time while I wrote; to Gae and Gerri, who ran a book-naming contest; to my husband, Jack, who once again, when I took on more than I could handle, was very calm and encouraging; and to my kids—Tom, Margaret, Lizzy, and Ann—who kept it all in perspective.

—Marion McCartney

To my sister, Ellen, who delivered at home, by midwife, and told me how great birth could be; to my midwife, Maureen Rayson, who delivered my daughter and proved that Ellen was right; to Peter, who stood beside me at every birth; to the beautiful end results of those births—my children, Nicolaas and Natalie and newborn Theodore (delivered at home by midwife), who grew inside me as this book grew to completion.

—Antonia van der Meer

Contents

Introduction

A Word from Marion McCartney, CNM

There are a lot of pregnancy books on the market these days, many of them written by obstetricians, but this one is different: it is written from the perspective of a certified nurse-midwife. As a mother of four, I think that childbirth should be a special, emotionally satisfying experience. As a nurse-midwife, I know it can be. I *chose* to be a nurse-midwife because the midwife is dedicated to keeping women well, as opposed to the physician, who is dedicated to healing sick people. In keeping with this philosophy, my approach to pregnancy and childbirth is less technological and just a little less conventional than an obstetrician's. The style of this book is very different from others written by doctors. I believe that women should be allowed to progress naturally through pregnancy and birth without fear, undue interference, or unnecessary rigidity. This type of birth can be achieved whether you use a doctor or midwife, whether you deliver in a hospital, birthing center, or at home. I've written this book to help you have a *normal*, happy birth.

I know that you are relatively inexperienced in this business, and you can easily become intimidated by all the choices you have ahead—where to deliver your baby, who should help you deliver your baby, what you should be eating, which prenatal tests to take, how you want your labor managed, and more.

Although these choices are all extremely important, the most critical factor in the outcome of your pregnancy is *you*. Your body is perfectly equipped to handle pregnancy and birth. Just consider the fact that without *intellectually* knowing how, you are able to grow a baby from a single cell into a complete human being with all of the highly complex organ systems that will ensure his or her survival and growth!

This fact has continued to amaze me throughout my fifteen years as a practicing nurse-midwife. The sheer miracle of birth is what drew me into this field. I remember the first delivery I ever watched. I was only a teenager, a high school student working as a nurse's aide in the local hospital. The idea of witnessing childbirth scared me, but when a doctor invited me in to see a delivery, I never thought to say no. It was a fantastic experience. As the baby's head came out, it turned toward me and there I was, staring at this perfect little face. With the next push, a baby girl was out and crying . . . and so was I! I was only seventeen, but I was hooked on childbirth, and destined to become a midwife years later. I have now delivered over six hundred babies, witnessed hundreds more deliveries, have given birth to four of my own children—and I'm *still* hooked on childbirth.

Before I became a midwife, I went to nursing school at Catholic University's School of Nursing. It was during my experiences there that I first began to see how much women needed coaching and support during labor and delivery—the kind of support that was rarely afforded them back then, the kind of support I want to offer you with this book. I began to teach childbirth classes to share what I had learned and to help prepare more women for the hours that would lie ahead of them at the birth. After I graduated from the midwifery school at Georgetown University, I delivered babies both at home and in the hospital. Then, in 1975, I founded Maternity Center Associates with other George-town graduates and we did home births and some hospital births.

In 1982 we added a free-standing birth center to our practice. A birth center stands apart from a hospital and offers total maternity care, including prenatal checkups, labor and birth management, and postpartum care, all in a warm, homelike atmosphere. There I care for pregnant women and deliver babies, with a team of other certified nurse-midwives. Because of the success of our center, I am often invited to speak about midwifery, childbirth legislation, malpractice, out-of-hospital births, and numerous other topics at gatherings across the country and on television.

But the most wonderful moments in my career as a nurse-midwife come at the birth of each baby I "catch." To experience the beginning of life fills me with awe. As often as I do it, childbirth never becomes commonplace. Babies are miraculous beings who are born with strong instincts for survival. I'd like to share with you my love of these beginnings and tell you how to give your baby the very best start possible. This book will give you an "insider's look" at obstetrics and midwifery today, plus invaluable advice and clear guidelines for a safe and natural pregnancy and birth. You need to be able to evaluate the pros and cons of new technologies and their alternatives in order to become an active participant in birth, not just a passive patient. An involved and informed approach makes for the healthiest delivery and leaves the new mother with feelings of increased self-esteem and self-respect—whether her labor was short or long, uncomplicated or medically assisted. Women want to be safe and feel relaxed when giving birth. Unfortunately, I think this is getting harder for them to do. I hope this book will make it a little easier.

In writing this book, I have drawn not only on my fifteen years of catching babies, but also on my association with wonderful obstetricians, nurses, and midwives, as well as grandmothers, aunts, sisters, and all the women who shared their stories and their births with me. I have learned from all of them. And I give all this to you.

—Marion McCartney

A Word from Antonia van der Meer

When I had my first baby I went into pregnancy with all the hopes and many of the insecurities that other first-time mothers have. Like other women, I spent a good deal of time picking an obstetrician with whom I felt comfortable and whose philosophies seemed to be in keeping with my own. Although I saw this doctor once a month, read books about pregnancy, and took childbirth classes, I never felt well prepared for the process that lay ahead. Like a secret recipe passed along by a wily friend, it all looked good but somehow something was missing. There was more information to be had, things I didn't know, and hadn't been told.

With my first labor pains I phoned my doctor. Twenty-four hours later, twelve of which were spent at the hospital, I gave birth to a beautiful seven-and-a-half-pound boy. But the experience didn't seem as beautiful as the baby I had just had. My caring doctor had become all business at the delivery, insisting that I stay in bed, popping in and out of the labor room every hour or so to "check" on my progress, which seemed slow and displeasing to him. He offered no suggestion for speeding my labor or strengthening my contractions other than a drug called Pitocin. By the time my son was born, I had survived arguments with an admitting nurse about mandatory enema and shaving (I was told I was risking serious infection by my refusal), an IV I didn't want, forceps I didn't think I needed, Pitocin which scared me, and an episiotomy I had hoped to avoid. Little had been done to make me feel I was in a supportive atmosphere. I felt somewhat bewildered and even betrayed by this approach to childbirth. Both my husband and baby were whisked away right after delivery and I was left alone in my room to "recover."

As distressing as parts of the childbirth experience were to me during that birth, I knew at the same time that it could be wonderful—I knew how much I loved the sight of my baby at birth. I wanted my second birth to be different. I wanted to use someone I trusted, a caregiver who would be supportive of my role. When I got pregnant a second time, I went to see another doctor—this time a woman—in the hope that her approach would be more enlightened. After waiting close to two hours in a beautifully appointed anteroom, I was ushered in through a maze of rooms and nurses' desks to see her. I asked about positions used during delivery, suggestions for avoiding episiotomies and how often she felt they were necessary, use of IVs and birthing rooms, and all those other good questions books tell us to ask potential caregivers on that first visit. Although she seemed nice enough and willing to "give my ideas a try," I decided that she was not for me. I didn't delude myself into thinking that I would be one of the 2 percent of her patients to avoid an episiotomy or the first to deliver without stirrups. I no longer wanted to fight the system and preferred to find a caregiver who routinely managed labor and birth the way I wanted it to be.

A little nervously I made an appointment with a midwife. I was nervous because I had been trained to trust only doctors with birth. I wondered, What if there were an emergency at birth? I concluded it was better to prepare for a normal birth with backup in case of a problem than to prepare for a problem birth with the outside chance of delivering normally. When I asked the midwife the same questions I had asked the doctor, I found someone who could do more than just give my way "a try." She was experienced in the type of birth I was searching for. She agreed that I could move about during labor and assume a less traditional position during delivery; she seemed confident that I would be able to avoid an episiotomy. What I found during the prenatal care, labor, and delivery of my second child was that missing ingredient that made childbirth wonderful in ways it had not been the first time. I found a caregiver who *urged* me to phone her between office visits when I had a worry or concern and who always listened to me, who told me everything she could about my body, my baby, and my health, and who believed in my ability to help myself and my baby through good nutrition, exercise, and understanding of the birth process. My second baby, a girl, was born in a spirit of joy, compassion, and trust, without an IV, without drugs, without forceps, without stirrups, without an episiotomy, without a tear.

I want to tell other women—whether they use a doctor or a midwife—that this is not another baby factory book. *You* are a very important person who deserves to know the missing ingredients so that your baby can grow within you and be delivered in the best way possible. Because my experience with a midwife was so positive, I went straight to one of the most well-respected midwives in the country, Marion McCartney, and asked her to write this book with me and share the midwife approach with all pregnant women. My coauthor and I cannot promise you an easy labor or a totally uncomplicated delivery, but with this book, we can help you have a better, more informed, less frightening experience.

—Antonia van der Meer

The
MIDWIFE'S
Pregnancy and
Childbirth
BOOK

1

Choosing a Caregiver

After the first tingle of delight when you discover you're pregnant comes a twinge of shock. What are you going to do now? Your thoughts turn almost immediately to finding a caregiver. You will want someone you like and trust, someone who understands your fears and concerns. But even more important, you will want someone whose views and attitudes about pregnancy and birth are similar to your own. Even if you've never been pregnant before, you probably already have strong feelings about what birth should be like. You may even know that there are many ways to manage labor and deliver babies: for example, with painkillers or without them, lying flat on a delivery table or sitting up in bed, in a hospital or at home. The caregiver you choose is very important because that person's biases, beliefs, habits, attitudes, and training will affect which of these routes your childbirth experience takes.

For women who perceive pregnancy as a natural event rather than an illness, and who seek a birth that is allowed to proceed without undue medical interference, a nurse-midwife is often the perfect choice. In fact, an increasing number of women today are seeking out nurse-midwives, like myself, for pregnancy care and childbirth management just for this reason. With a nurse-midwife, women are able to give birth safely in a supportive atmosphere of mutual respect. Many of my clients tell me that they prefer a nurse-midwife to a doctor because midwives see pregnancy and birth not as a serious medical condition but as a normal and beautiful process. I think what appeals to these women most is the nurse-midwife's emphasis on education and the spirit of cooperation that exists between mother and midwife in the birthing process. Midwives have the time to listen to a mother's concerns and to educate her about pregnancy and childbirth. Much of my office time is spent talking with the prospective parents, grandparents, and siblings about the coming birth. Whether or not you ultimately choose to use a nurse-midwife, you will still benefit from the natural, caring approach I offer you in this book. My advice is based on years spent listening to mothers and their families.

Choosing a nurse-midwife is a very important first step in ensuring the type of birth you want to have. With all the choices out there, you have a right to have your baby your way.

The Certified Nurse-Midwife

I am often told at the first meeting with an expectant woman: "You don't look at all like what I expected." This statement reflects many of the misconceptions the public has about certified nurse-midwives. People picture either gray-haired grannies with little formal education or hippies left over from the 1960s. This is far from the truth for today's certified nurse-midwife.

There are about 3,000 certified nurse-midwives like myself currently at work in the United States. We are health-care professionals, registered nurses (RNs) with advanced training (one to two years or more) in pregnancy, childbirth, gynecology, and family planning. After successfully completing an accredited university program and passing national boards (administered by the American College of Nurse-Midwives), an RN becomes a *certified nurse-midwife*, or CNM. She or he is then licensed by the state as an RN and a CNM.

To avoid confusion, I would like to make clear at the outset that in some states a person can be a midwife without being a certified *nurse*-midwife. This person is known as a *professional midwife*. A professional midwife is licensed by the state but she is not a nurse. She has attended a program recognized by the state that includes extensive hands-on experience with mothers and babies. The professional midwife delivers babies primarily at home. You may also come across an *unlicensed midwife*. Unlicensed midwives come from a wide variety of backgrounds. They may have extensive educational training or very little at all. Without a license to ensure some standard of practice, it is very difficult to determine which of these lay midwives are good and which are not. Unlicensed midwives are illegal in most states. I believe it is safest to use licensed midwives only, and preferably certified nurse-midwives. You should always ask whether you are speaking with a nurse-midwife, a professional midwife, or an unlicensed midwife. In the United States most midwives are nurse-midwives. When I refer to midwives in this book, I'm referring to *certified nurse-midwives*.

Is a certified nurse-midwife a safe alternative to an obstetrician? Yes! Nurse-midwives are very well educated, have appropriate clinical skills, and know what to do in a wide variety of circumstances and difficulties. They can provide a woman with the same quality of care as obstetricians, assuming a basically normal birth. A patient who uses a nurse-midwife need not see a physician as long as the course of her pregnancy and birth remains essentially normal. For serious complications of pregnancy and birth, a physician's skills are needed. For this reason, a midwife always has an arrangement with a backup physician. In our practice, each woman visits the backup doctor during her pregnancy so that a feeling of mutual trust and understanding can develop. If a serious complication does occur, the nurse-midwife remains involved in the patient's care even if she doesn't actually do the delivery. The transition between caregivers is smooth and orderly, so the woman gets the best of both worlds. She can have a nurse-midwife who strives to keep her healthy and well educated, and an obstetrician who can step in if complications arise. Each health-care person contributes his or her expertise as needed.

This brings us to the question of *what is normal?* The definition of "normal" can of course be debated. No pregnancy and birth are totally uneventful. For this reason, the term *essentially normal* is used to describe the scope of a nurse-midwife's practice. Nurse-midwives are well trained to handle the things that can (and do) go wrong during labor and childbirth. Nurse-midwives have the knowledge, judgment, and skill to perform many medical interventions, from an episiotomy (a cut to widen the vaginal opening) and pudendal block (a form of pain relief) to intubation and resuscitation of the newborn. They are educated, however, to promote the *natural process of childbirth*, keeping the patient informed of all decisions and staying within the limits of safety as determined by the patient's medical condition. A nurse-midwife will not usually handle independently serious complications such as a breech delivery (when the baby is feet- or bottom-first), a pregnant woman with diabetes, or a woman carrying multiple fetuses. Happily, most serious complications are quite rare. At least 80 percent of all women need no unusual medical assistance for the pregnancy, labor, or birth. Of the remaining 20 percent, most can be identified as at risk for certain problems long before labor begins.

A Brief History of Midwifery and Obstetrics

American midwifery is as old as our nation. Among the first women settlers were midwives. These women were accorded special privileges in return for their work, such as free housing, land, and food. By the 1800s, physicians decided to practice midwifery, and the male doctor began to replace the female midwife on the birthing scene. Obstetrics as a specialty really didn't exist back then. At the beginning of the nineteenth century the first textbook on obstetrics was published, but not until 1930 was obstetrics an established specialty in medical schools. In the early 1900s, the vast majority of deliveries were still conducted at home (by physicians) and hospitals were not set up for births or even for emergency obstetrical care. There was essentially no prenatal care before 1920. Medical care was confined to the birth itself.

Nurse-midwifery sprang to new life in the United States during the 1930s as a way to reach pregnant women far removed from big-city medical care. It began in eastern Kentucky, where women in rural areas could, for the first time, benefit from the services of a childbirth expert. Nurse-midwives of the Frontier Nursing Service gave prenatal care, delivered babies, immunized children and adults, and provided health care. The infant and maternal mortality rate dropped dramatically due to these early leaders in nurse-midwifery. Somewhat like the Pony Express, midwives delivered come rain or shine.

Nurse-midwives, however, were not widely used in the United States until the late 1960s, when women began looking for more control over their own health care. Today, midwives serve patients throughout the country, delivering babies at home, in hospitals, and in birthing centers. Their patients come from all walks of life, all income and educational levels. In many European countries, midwives are the predominant providers of obstetrical care. (In Norway, for example, almost 96 percent of women use midwives for prenatal care and delivery.) Although in the United States an MD is more common, times are changing. The World Health Organization has stated that midwives ought to be the primary caregivers for normal childbearing women. The number of midwife-assisted births is on the rise, as parents look for more inclusive, less intrusive maternity and childbirth care. The number of midwife-assisted births has tripled from just 30,000 to over 100,000 in the past ten years and will probably continue to rise.

Why So Many Women Are Using Midwives Today

There are many reasons why women are turning to midwives in increasing numbers.

• Women are increasingly confident that they can give birth without unnecessary medical intervention. Many women are beginning to believe that medicine and invasive techniques are used too often in childbirth.

Midwives view childbirth as a *natural* process. Technological intervention is practiced only when necessary. Midwives agree that high-tech intervention has its place but argue that it has never been proved that it produces better outcomes for *normal* women. Midwives are experienced in normal, natural births, and know how to manage them. Doctors are experienced in pathological, or problem, births, and are often less interested in the management of a normal birth.

• Women are becoming assertive, well-informed consumers with their own views of how a normal birth should progress.

A midwife's approach to pregnancy is usually less dogmatic and rigid than a doctor's. A midwife is not threatened by a woman who is educated about her own body, pregnancy, and childbirth.

• Women want to deliver safely in an atmosphere of mutual respect.

A midwife-assisted birth is just as safe as a birth by an obstetrician, or OB. In fact, in a 1986 report of the American College of Nurse-Midwives Foundation, which reviewed available studies on the safety of nurse-midwife care, the studies indicated that "CNM care resulted in similar or better outcomes of pregnancy for mothers and infants when compared with physician care in the same area."

• Women sometimes prefer to be cared for by women.

Midwives are almost always women. OBs are almost always men.

• Most women today want to learn as much as they can about their bodies and the work of childbirth that lies ahead.

Nurse-midwives emphasize preparedness for their patients—through nutrition, exercise, and childbirth education.

• Women want pregnancy and childbirth to be psychologically positive experiences.

Nurse-midwives realize the importance of a woman's emotional state, social background, and behavioral factors as they come into play in prenatal care, childbirth, and delivery. They spend a great deal of time with their patients, explaining and teaching. They spend time talking with their patients so that women don't feel they've been rushed in and out to accommodate a fifteen-minute time slot. There is no assembly-line approach to care.

• Women need and appreciate personal support during labor and birth—support that reduces anxiety and increases their ability to cope with pain.

Midwives labor-sit; they are committed to being with their patients during the crucial phases of labor and provide encouragement, support, and coping mechanisms for the laboring woman.

• Some women want to have husbands, children, or other relatives at the birth.

Midwives believe that birth is a family event. Significant family members, even children, are not excluded, assuming the woman wants them at the birth.

• Many women prefer that medical interventions be suggested on an individual-case basis, rather than be applied to all laboring women.

In midwifery each patient is treated as an individual and decisions are made about her unique situation. There is no one set of rules by which all pregnant women are expected to perform. For example, a midwife will probably apply practical experience and common sense rather than set a strict time limit on the pushing phase of the delivery.

• There has been increasing interest in the possibility of avoiding one of the most common birth interventions: the episiotomy (a cut to enlarge the vaginal opening). Women often want to avoid an episiotomy because it is intrusive, uncomfortable, and possibly unnecessary surgery.

Nurse-midwives are adept at avoiding episiotomies and tears in the vaginal area at the delivery. Most obstetricians tell their patients that an episiotomy is a normal part of all first-time deliveries. Nurse-midwives don't agree. They perform this surgical incision only when they deem it medically necessary and unavoidable. Instead, they practice methods of avoiding the incision *and* usually avoid serious tearing of the perineum as well.

• Women are beginning to focus on the importance of *their* role at the birth, as opposed to the doctor's.

Nurse-midwives see their job as assisting the mother in delivering a baby; doctors often view their job simply as delivering the baby.

• A number of women are concerned about the high costs of obstetrical care.

Normal pregnancies can be managed by nurse-midwives in birth centers for about 40 percent of the cost of obstetric care, according to a 1980 study reported by the American College of Nurse-Midwives (ACNM). A 1982 study by the Health Insurance Association of America concluded that the use of midwives can decrease the costs of having babies due to the normally shorter length of hospital stays. In addition, the midwife's less technical approach to normal birth is less costly while capable of achieving the same good maternal and infant outcomes. The U.S. Office of Technology Assessment concluded in a 1986 paper that "Given that the quality of care provided by CNMs within their areas of competence is equivalent to the quality of comparable services provided by physicians, using CNMs rather than physicians to provide certain services would appear to be cost-effective."

• Most women today are concerned about the alarmingly high rates of cesarean births in the United States.
A greater use of midwives seems to correlate with lower C-section rates. In a report of 2,600 women in the north central Bronx, published by Doris Haire, president of the American Foundation for Maternal and Child Health, in 1979 nurse-midwives delivered 83 percent of the women, both high- and low-risk, and had excellent outcomes. The C-section rate was only 9 percent, compared with a rate of about 20 percent nationwide at the same time. (Today's C-section rate is 25 percent.) Even though as many as two-thirds of the mothers were considered high-risk or at risk for problems, as many as 88 percent had normal spontaneous vaginal births by midwives.

• Some women are interested in giving birth outside the hospital.
Midwives offer their patients a choice of birthing places: in the home, in the hospital, and in a free-standing birth center.

• Women want caregivers they trust and respect.
There is a very high rate of patient satisfaction reported with midwifery care. Nurse-midwives tend to spend more time with patients, to be more attentive to their needs and worries. Midwives are trained to be good listeners who value their patients' feelings. In a study done by the University of Mississippi Medical Center, nurse-midwife clients kept 94 percent of their appointments as compared with the staff physicians' patients, who kept only 80 percent of their appointments. Nurse-midwives also have a very low lawsuit rate (6 percent of all CNMs have been sued for malpractice as compared with 70 percent of all obstetricians), another measure of patient satisfaction.

When it comes to *your* prenatal care and birth, how would a midwife really differ from a doctor? To help you further understand some of the distinctions between the two, consider some of these comparisons:

A doctor might say: "It's easier to deliver a baby when the woman is on her back on a delivery table."
A midwife would say: "It's easiest for the mother to deliver in the position most comfortable for *her*—squatting, sitting, lying on her side."

A doctor might say: "Ninety-eight percent of all first-time mothers need an episiotomy."
A midwife would say: "Episiotomies are most often unnecessary interventions. They can be safely avoided even for the first-time mother."

A doctor might say: "Let's put in the IV just in case you get tired and need it."
A midwife would say: "Let's not use the IV unless you get tired. To make sure you don't run out of energy, you should drink lots of sweetened beverages."

A doctor might say: "If you don't dilate in the next two hours, we'll do a cesarean."
A midwife would say: "You're making slow progress. Let's get you up and walk around and see if that helps."

A doctor might say: "I know it's painful. Why not take an epidural?"
A midwife would say: "I know it's painful . . . let's work through the contractions together to get this baby born. For now, let's also try the Jacuzzi for relief from back pain, okay?"

A doctor might say: "The baby can spend the night in the nursery so you can rest."
A midwife would say: "Perhaps you'd like to keep the baby with you so you can nurse on demand."

These comparisons highlight just a few of the differences between most doctors and most nurse-midwives. Unquestionably, there are times and situations when an MD is essential, but for a normal delivery either practitioner is appropriate and a midwife may be preferable. If you cannot locate a midwife in your area, look for a doctor whose style and way of thinking are similar to a midwife's. Philosophies and practices should be investigated, discussed, and weighed so you can decide who is best for you.

Other Medical Specialists

If you cannot find or do not wish to use a nurse-midwife, you may choose an obstetrician, perinatologist, or family practitioner. An *obstetrician* is a medical doctor who has had four years of residency training in obstetrics and gynecology. The focus of his or her training is on pathology and problems in childbirth. Obstetricians practice almost exclusively in hospitals. A few deliver babies in birth centers or at home. A *perinatologist* is an obstetrician with a specialty in high-risk pregnancies and births. A *family practitioner* is a doctor who most resembles the traditional general practitioner of years gone by. He or she is an MD who has done a residency in general family medicine including obstetrics and gynecology. Family practice physicians are usually restricted from performing many high-risk births (such as C-sections) and must refer certain patients to obstetricians, as do certified nurse-midwives.

Where to Find a Practitioner

There are a number of places where you can begin your search for a nurse-midwife or doctor. As you speak to these sources, you'll start to hear a name or two repeatedly mentioned. These are people you should interview. Be cautious in your search for the right person. Don't accept a name blindly; you'll want to talk with the midwife or doctor before you choose. Rely on your own instincts and on what makes you comfortable. To find some names:

1. Ask childbirth educators for referrals. They're in the Yellow Pages. Even though you don't know them, they will readily

give recommendations. Childbirth educators hear about all the nurse-midwives and doctors in the area and have a good sense of who is "into" natural childbirth and who isn't, who's good and who isn't. Childbirth-education groups often have midwives and doctors on their boards whom they can recommend to you.

2. Call La Leche League for names of nurse-midwives and doctors. The international organization for the support of breast-feeding is located at 9616 Minneapolis Avenue, Franklin Park, IL 60131 (312–455–7730). Or call your local chapter, listed in the phone book.

3. Speak to your current gynecologist (if he or she is not an obstetrician) or other family doctor. Explain that you are looking for a nurse-midwife or a doctor with a philosophy similar to a midwife's.

4. If you have a friend who is a nurse, ask her to put you in touch with a labor-and-delivery nurse, who will certainly know everyone's reputation and who's good at what!

5. Pediatricians are often good sources. Tell them what kind of person and practice you're searching for.

6. Call the American College of Nurse-Midwives in Washington, D.C., and ask for the names of CNMs in your area.

7. Call a hospital. Some hospitals have referral services. Again, it may help to ask for the type of practitioner you want. Ask specifically for a midwife if you prefer one.

8. Read articles and books about childbirth. You may find names of certain experts near you.

9. Listen to other women. Ask them which midwives or obstetricians they liked. Try to get a recommendation from a woman whose attitudes and views about childbirth are similar to yours.

10. Contact a teaching hospital if you are looking for a high-risk specialist.

How to Make the Final Decision

This is your body, your pregnancy, your baby. To find the best person to fill this very important role of adviser, protector, and caregiver, begin your search early. Don't panic, though, if you're already two, three, or even four months pregnant and still searching. It would be ideal if the first person you saw was the right one for you, but this is not always realistic. It is wise, however, to try to settle the question as soon as possible so you can receive continuous, unified care and advice from one person.

Interviewing these people takes time and often costs money as well, but it's worth it. Bring your spouse, friend, or relative for moral support and to ask questions you may feel too intimidated to ask. Make a written list of the issues that are important to you so you won't forget. A spouse or friend can also help to give a second opinion. Once there:

1. Observe the office environment: Is it relaxed or formal? Extremely busy? Impersonal or warm? Orderly or muddled?
2. Is there information about pregnancy and childbirth readily available? Is there a lending library? Brochures, pamphlets, etc.?
3. Is the staff friendly and helpful or distant and close-mouthed? Do people introduce themselves? Do they make eye contact when they talk to you?
4. How are the phones answered? Much of your contact with the office may be by phone, when you call in with questions, concerns, even possible emergencies. Are calls between visits encouraged or frowned upon? Who handles the calls? Are phone calls dealt with the way you'd like them to be?
5. Do you feel like an adult when you speak to the midwife or doctor? Does everyone use the same title? Or do you address the physician as "Dr. Rider" while she uses your first name to address you?
6. Are your questions welcome or are they answered defensively, even hostilely?

7. Is medical information such as your charts and test results shared openly with you? At the Maternity Center, our clients read their charts at every visit. In fact, the first thing they do when they arrive is pick up their chart, weigh themselves, and fill in the data. (This is unusual but indicates that the office is open about communication with the patient.)

8. Is this a group practice? How many midwives or doctors are in the practice? Do they have an "on call" schedule? Most group practices rotate the "on call" status so that when you go into labor you may not actually be cared for by the particular midwife or doctor you chose and know best. On the positive side, the group practice ensures that you won't have an exhausted doctor or CNM at the delivery. To ease the transition, group practices usually insist that the pregnant woman have appointments with all the practitioners in the group. This way, she gets to know them all before the delivery. The midwife or doctor you choose may instead work alone. The benefit to a solo practice is knowing that *this* is the face you'll see at the birth. Find out who the backup practitioner will be in case of this caregiver's illness or vacation.

9. Who is the backup doctor? If you use a nurse-midwife, she will have an arrangement with an obstetrician who can step in to handle high-risk problems of pregnancy and birth. Can you meet him or her? (You may wish to, as there is always the chance that your care will end up in his or her hands.)

How to Ask Important Questions

All books tell you to ask questions politely, without insulting the practitioner or making him or her defensive. But most people don't know *how* to ask difficult questions. Most midwives expect questions and are used to answering them openly. Many doctors, however, are used to being authority figures, and it's possible that your questions will make them feel defensive, especially if the subject is sensitive. Don't get nervous. Relax. Smile. You are just getting information. There *are* ways to ask about C-section rates without offending anyone. Here's how to best couch some tough questions that you really do need answers to.

GENERAL ATTITUDE

• "I appreciate your taking time to talk to me. It's very important to me to get general ideas about a practice before starting out. Can you describe your philosophy of care for pregnancy and birth?"
• "Can you describe how a typical, very normal labor usually goes?"

USE OF PAINKILLERS

• "I know many women like myself think they want natural childbirth and then get into labor and have second thoughts and possibly end up with epidurals. How often does this happen in your practice?" (Try to get a percentage figure.)
• "If I were experiencing a lot of pain during delivery, what might you suggest we try besides an epidural or other drug?"

DELIVERY POSITIONS

• "I have heard that many women find that vertical positions (sitting, squatting) are easier for labor and delivery. Do you find this to be true? In your experience, what are the most favorable delivery positions? Which do your patients most often use?"

EPISIOTOMIES

• "I'd like to understand the reasons behind the use of episiotomies. Could you explain when they are necessary and why? How many first-time mothers are given episiotomies? Which, if any, of your patients do not need one? Is this by chance or are there ways to prepare for delivery without a cut?"

C-SECTION RATE

• "I'm interested in knowing more about C-sections. I know they are much safer than in the past and are often used for fetal distress. What has your experience been? What is the rate at the hospital where you deliver? What is your rate overall including high- and low-risk women?"

BREAST-FEEDING

• "I'd like more information about breast-feeding. I've heard most women can breast-feed. In your experience do they? What influences their decision to switch to bottles?"

• "Do most mothers in your practice end up breast-feeding only, bottle-feeding only, or a combination of both?"

BONDING

• "After delivery I understand it's important to keep the baby warm and for the parents to spend time bonding with the baby. If everything is normal what usually happens?"

• "Is there required nursery time for the baby after birth?"

• "Is rooming-in available at the hospital where you practice? How does it work? How do you feel about it?"

By making questions open-ended, it is easier to assess the attitude of the midwife or doctor. Remember, attitudes are the most important measure of the person. Attitudes influence a person's decisions. If, for example, the practitioner feels that most women are tired after the birth and that bonding has been blown out of proportion by the media, you might expect that he or she will not encourage rooming-in and may not use a hospital where it is comfortably allowed. Credentials are easy to verify, but attitudes are more difficult to pinpoint.

Don't overlook answers you don't like. Keep them in mind when you make your decision. Believe the statistics you are given. If a doctor you interview says that he finds 98 percent of his first-time mothers need an episiotomy, don't kid yourself into thinking that you'll be one of the 2 percent he doesn't cut. Face the fact that his beliefs and attitudes are what they are and base your decision on the realities of the situation, not what you wish it to be. Keep looking until you find the answers you want to hear.

2

Where Should I Have
My Baby?

Today, women have more than one option available to them when it comes to birthing locations: home, birth center, and hospital. Each provides a very distinct atmosphere with very different resources. Often, the choice of your location goes hand in hand with your choice of practitioner. One nurse-midwife may deliver only at home, another nurse-midwife may work only in a birth center, a third only at a hospital. So if you have already chosen a caregiver, the decision of where to have the baby may be made for you. If where you give birth is very important to you—if, for example, a home birth is what you really want, or if you feel you must be at a particular teaching hospital—you may have to work backward by choosing the caregiver *after* you've chosen the location.

In this chapter, I give you the facts about each location, but I start with a firsthand view of a birth in all three places: at home, in a birth center, and in a hospital. I have delivered babies in all three settings. My personal stories begin each section and should give you a feel for what it is like to have a child in each location.

The Home-Birth Experience

The phone rang and woke me around 4:00 A.M. It was Sara, one of my patients, and she was in labor with her fourth baby. I got up and looked out the window. It had been snowing during the night and big white flakes were still falling as I dressed and drove to Sara's house in Maryland. I had delivered her three other children, all born at home, and was happy to be on my way to "catch" another.

Sara answered the door and we both remarked on how fortunate it was that she always seemed to go into labor when I was on call. The children were all still asleep and the house was quiet. Lenny, her husband, was in the kitchen, calling a friend who had agreed to come over and help with the other children during the birth.

I took my delivery equipment into the bedroom and unpacked the emergency equipment I might need for mother and baby, such as oxygen tank and drugs to control bleeding after birth. I saw that Sara had already set up her own home-birth supplies. There was a waterproof cover under the sheets of her king-size bed. She had disposable underpads, some paper towels handy, and a copy of her prenatal chart. Her hospital bag was packed and sitting on a chair in the corner. (Mothers need to have this ready just in case a problem arises that would necessitate a move to the hospital.) I also checked to make sure she had filled out her preadmission form to the hospital (she had).

I examined Sara and told her she was five centimeters dilated. With a Doppler we listened to the baby's heartbeat through a couple of contractions. The heartbeat sounded good, meaning the baby was tolerating the labor well. Then it was off to the kitchen for a cup of coffee and a phone call to the birth assistant, a nurse who frequently helps with home births. She told me she'd be there within the hour. There is always a veteran labor-and-delivery nurse at a home birth. An extra pair of experienced hands on the premises is invaluable, even lifesaving. I sat down and began filling out Sara's labor chart, carefully recording all of the mother's and baby's vital signs and the mother's progress in labor. I was just finishing up my first notations when Sara and Lenny's oldest child came into the room. An eight-year-old girl, she was for the moment more interested in school closings than in the arrival of her new sibling. We listened to the radio announcements together as the snow continued to fall. It was just 6:00 A.M. Soon all three children were up, eating cereal, watching the snow, listening to the radio, and eyeing this visiting midwife. When the school closing was finally announced, there were whoops of joy from the three kids. A friend of the family had arrived to take care of the children so Sara and Lenny would be free to cope with the labor. The children were aged eight, four, and two, and they couldn't wait to get outside and play in the snow.

Barbara, the nurse, arrived around seven, and we took turns monitoring the baby's heart while Sara walked around the house in labor. Sara needed very little help from either of us. She was coping beautifully with the labor, and she and Lenny made a wonderful team. For the next two hours we sipped coffee, listened to the baby, watched the snow fall, and waited. Labor sitting has taught me the virtues of relaxing while waiting. I have learned to be patient, sit back and observe the parents' behavior. It seemed Sara would soon be ready to push.

The kids and baby-sitter began to make a birthday cake for this new arrival. All three children—even the two-year-old—were "helping."

Sara and Lenny went to the bedroom. Barbara and I followed. Labor was progressing rapidly now. Sara lay on her side on the bed, doing Lamaze breathing while Lenny rubbed her back. She continued to look amazingly relaxed even when the contractions were back-to-back. When she had the urge to push, Lenny sat behind her on the bed and supported her in his arms. The children waited in the kitchen or family room. The older girl had been coming in to check on things every ten minutes or so. Then, I suppose, she reported back to the troops outside.

With the next push, Sara's water broke and gushes of clear, warm, amniotic fluid splashed everywhere. I quickly changed the disposable pad under her to make a comfortable dry spot. With the next contraction she pushed out a healthy baby girl with a shock of black hair who started crying as soon as she felt the room air on her wet skin. Sara reached down and picked her up from my gloved hands, cradling her in her arms and comforting her. Barbara covered them with warm blankets that had been kept next to the heating pad. Lenny and Sara began to talk about who the baby looked like—her sister's eyes, Grandpa's strong chin, and so on. I clamped the cord and Lenny cut it. I collected some extra cord blood for Rh studies. Sara was Rh-negative; if the baby was Rh-positive, Sara would need an injection of RhoGAM within seventy-two hours of the birth. We stored that blood in the refrigerator and Lenny was instructed to bring it into the hospital lab later that day.

After Sara delivered the placenta and we put another set of clean pads under her, I began to pack up my equipment. I had used only routine items during the delivery (sterile gloves, bulb syringe to suction the baby's nose and mouth, cord clamp), so everything I hadn't used went back into my two bags.

Without much hesitation, Sara and Lenny named their new baby Alexandra and then called all the children in to meet this beautiful new addition to the family. Sara had the children sit on the bed, one at a time, to hold the new baby. We had each one sit cross-legged in the center of the bed with a pillow in his or her lap. That made it possible for even the two-year-old to hold the baby alone and to feel part of this family celebration. As Lenny took pictures of each one of them, the happiness and excitement in the room was tangible. Sara nursed the baby while Lenny helped the children decorate the birthday cake. There were just a few loose ends left for me to tie up. The birth certificate still had to be filled out. Food and drinks were being taken up to Sara (women who've just delivered are often very hungry and deserve a good meal after all their hard work). After she had eaten something, we helped her into the bathroom to shower and then changed the sheets on the bed. The old sheets were stripped off and soaked in cold water and ammonia to remove the bloodstains. The baby was weighed using a portable fish-hook scale the nurse had brought with her. I gave the baby a complete newborn physical, administered state-required eye drops, gave the vitamin K shot, and called the pediatrician to arrange a visit within the next twenty-four hours. Barbara checked Sara often for any bleeding, took her vital signs, and we both reviewed postpartum instructions with the parents.

Just as I was about ready to leave, almost two hours after the birth, the kids and Lenny came in with the cake and one candle. They sang a chorus of "Happy Birthday" to baby Alexandra. We all toasted the birth with champagne for the adults, milk for the kids, and then it was time for me to head home. Barbara stayed on for another two hours or so to make sure mother and baby were just fine.

Almost ten inches of snow was on the ground now, and traveling back to my D.C. home wasn't a snap, but it was certainly easier for me to get to Sara than it would have been for her to travel on a day like this! Luckily, I was prepared with a twenty-five-pound bag of sand and a shovel in the back of my station wagon.

I felt very close to them all and took great pleasure in providing health care to a woman who believed that home births were best for her and her family.

The Home Birth

There are many advantages to doing things the old-fashioned way. Having your baby born in the comfort and privacy of your own home can be warm and wonderful. There are also some risks and disadvantages that should be considered carefully before you make a decision.

Women considering a home birth should be carefully screened to determine the safety of such a decision in their particular case. Home birth is for women who are considered to be "low-risk," meaning there is no reason to assume that the birth will be anything but normal. These women should have no heart disease or diabetes and no family history of genetic disorders. Multiple births should not be handled at home. Breech and premature births should also be conducted in a hospital setting instead. Even if a woman meets all the medical criteria for a home birth, there is always the chance that a problem will arise that cannot be dealt with at home; she may have to be moved to a hospital in the event of an unforeseen complication. For this reason, the woman should live within a reasonable distance of a hospital (so that a C-section can be started within thirty minutes of an emergency situation). Nurse-midwives who deliver at home, however, are adept at handling many common problems, such as resuscitation of newborns (who sometimes need some extra help getting started), repair of episiotomies under local anesthesia, use of drugs to control bleeding after delivery, and the use of IV fluids.

Are planned home births safe for low-risk women? Yes. Some people think they may be even safer than hospital births! In the Netherlands, where about 40 percent of the babies are born at home, the rate of perinatal mortality (babies born dead or who die shortly after birth) is one of the lowest in the world. A study done by the British Birth Survey (1970) showed that babies born in a hospital were five times more likely to have breathing difficulties than babies born at home. In a study of 5,000 home births in Holland, only a few deaths occurred; and researchers concluded that of these, none could have been prevented if the birth had been in a hospital. Planned home births produced babies with a higher birth weight in another British study reported in a 1984 lecture.

ADVANTAGES OF A HOME BIRTH

1. For some women, their own turf is the most comfortable place to deliver, surrounded by familiar objects and family members.
2. A home birth allows the most individuality and flexibility.
3. At home, you can avoid the often routine interventions practiced in a hospital such as IV, electronic fetal monitoring, enemas, epidurals, etc.

4. The cost of a home birth is less than that of a hospital birth.

5. There is no need to uproot yourself and move to a hospital or birth center; the caregiver comes to *you*.

6. The midwife is a guest in your home.

7. If you have other children, they do not feel upset by the disappearance of their mother, who then returns days later with a new baby. They are able to experience the birth of the sibling as a natural extension of family life. If the parents wish, they can allow the children in the room for the birth, something that is rarely an option in a hospital.

8. There are no admissions procedures, no forms, no set policies.

9. You can wear your own nightgown or T-shirt or even nothing at all if you feel most comfortable that way.

10. There are no uninvited doctors, residents, or nurses popping in to view the birth.

11. You feel free to move around, eat, and drink if you please.

12. Drugs are not used, except to repair tears or stop heavy bleeding after delivery.

13. Your labor is more likely to progress naturally without interference.

14. The baby won't be taken away from you after birth. There's no mandatory "nursery time." Breast-feeding is often easier to establish without this interruption or the possibility of a nurse offering a bottle.

15. Your husband may feel more involved in the birth when it takes place in your own home. He can wear his regular clothes and won't feel so much like a trespasser in the maternity ward.

16. The baby is less likely to get an infection. Hospitals are filled with sick people and other people's germs, and the hospital staff must be constantly on guard against cross-infection. At home, your baby is exposed only to the immediate family.

17. You don't have to share a room with other mothers and babies, as you might in a hospital. You have your peace and your privacy.

DISADVANTAGES OF A HOME BIRTH

1. You may have to be moved to a hospital during labor if there are warning signs of maternal or fetal distress. The facilities for emergencies are not down the hall; they are a car ride away.
2. The move to a hospital can be upsetting to parents both because it signals problems and because plans for a special and personal birth are now so radically altered.
3. You may feel nervous waiting for your caregiver to arrive and prefer to have the responsibility of getting yourself to the caregiver on time.
4. You may feel uncomfortable with the thought of having your other children around or nervous that they will hear you shout or scream, even if they are kept out of the way in another room.
5. Even though home birth sounds good, you may feel it's too unconventional or that it seems somehow unsafe to deliver at home. This uneasiness may slow down your labor.
6. At home, you won't have the twenty-four-hour hospital services at your beck and call (food, nursing, infant care).

Questions to Ask About Home Birth

You should speak with a home-birth practitioner before making a final decision about home birth. Here are some questions you may want to get answered before you go ahead with a home birth:

How close is the nearest hospital to my home?
The nearest hospital should be close enough that you can be on the delivery table and getting a C-section within thirty minutes.

How would I be transported there? By ambulance or by car?
Both should be available. If time is of the essence, you should be transported by ambulance.

How receptive is the hospital to handling an emergency that arises out of a delivery begun at home?
Your midwife will know how welcoming the hospital will be, and she can tell you about her experiences there. The hospital will not, of course, turn you away, but some parents feel very uncomfortable delivering in a hospital that looks upon home-birth transfers disapprovingly.

Does my midwife have privileges at this hospital?
You have a right to know who will be delivering your baby in case of a move to the hospital. Could the midwife at your home birth complete the delivery at the hospital using the hospital's facilities? If not, who will? Is it her backup physician or the hospital obstetrician on duty at the time of the crisis?

If I am moved to a hospital, will my midwife stay with me even if she cannot do deliveries there?
The answer to this question should be yes. She should meet the obstetrician with you so that she can talk with him or her and help establish a plan of care. It is also comforting for you simply to know whether she will remain as a support person for you.

Who assists the CNM at a home birth?
The midwife should not attempt to deliver your baby alone. A certified nurse-midwife should always work with an experienced birth assistant (usually a labor-and-delivery nurse) at a home birth. Two pairs of hands are essential. For example, if the baby has to be transported to a hospital, one of the team must go with the baby while the other remains with the mother.

What supplies and equipment do I need to have at home?
The midwife will supply you with a complete list, including such items as a thermometer, disposable bed pads, a dozen receiving blankets, rubbing alcohol, a baby scale, a preadmission form to the nearest hospital, a packed suitcase in case of a transfer there, etc.

What supplies and equipment will the midwife bring?
The midwife will bring sterile gloves, a local painkiller such as

Xylocaine, suture material to repair a tear, sterile cord clamps, sterile scissors, equipment to suction out the baby's nose and mouth, vitamin K for newborn injection, silver nitrate or erythromycin for baby's eyes, tubes to collect cord blood, oxygen tank, IV fluids, stethoscope, blood pressure cuff, drugs to control postpartum hemorrhage, Doppler and fetoscope to listen to the baby's heartbeat.

What types of emergencies can be handled at home and which would prompt a move to a hospital?
Although long and even painful labors and births can be handled well at home, true medical emergencies cannot. A midwife should move you to a hospital in the event of maternal high blood pressure, fetal distress, abnormal bleeding, breech birth, or thick meconium found in the amniotic fluid. You should also be moved if you are not progressing in labor, as drugs to speed labor can be given only in the hospital. At home, a midwife can handle resuscitation of the newborn with intubation and oxygen, and the control of maternal postpartum hemorrhaging. If the bleeding cannot be well controlled or the baby's breathing not easily stabilized, the midwife will then transfer the mother and/or baby to the hospital.

Do I have to preregister at a particular hospital just in case I need to go there?
It is a good idea to preregister with the hospital so that you don't get caught in red tape during an admission.

Who will examine the baby after birth? Who will administer the necessary eye drops, injections? Do I need to contact a pediatrician?
Your midwife will examine the baby and administer the injections and eye drops. The midwife will not leave if there are *any* signs of newborn distress. A pediatrician should also see the baby within forty-eight hours of the birth. You will need to contact a pediatrician before your delivery. Your midwife can refer you to a pediatrician if you don't already have someone in mind.

Who fills out the birth certificate?
The midwife should do this.

The Birth Center Experience

Claire and Matthew called me at the Maternity Center and wanted to come in during office hours to be checked. Claire had been having irregular contractions for several hours. I told her to come and within a half hour she had arrived at our small, two-story house on a quiet street near the hospital. Normally, she would go downstairs to one of the prenatal examination rooms, but this time I led her straight upstairs to one of the three bedrooms we use for labor and delivery. We picked up her chart on the way. There were no admitting forms or any other papers to sign. She had had a bloody show, meaning the mucus plug was coming out of the cervix, but the contractions were irregular and mild and she was only about three centimeters dilated. After discussing the pros and cons, I stretched her cervix for her in the hopes of stimulating stronger contractions and then advised her to walk around and drink plenty of high-calorie fluids. Rather than pace the halls of the birth center, she and Matthew left and took a stroll around a nearby mall, window-shopping for Christmas presents. Back at home, their two little boys were anxiously awaiting news of the baby's arrival.

When Claire returned to the center around noon, she was four centimeters dilated and contractions were picking up. She and Matthew went upstairs and settled into the corner bedroom, the one we call the "heart room" because the wallpaper has tiny hearts of red, blue, and yellow. There's blue carpeting on the floor. A four-poster mahogany bed with a white bedspread and tons of comfy pillows takes up the center of the room. There are two windows with white tie-back curtains and a large mahogany dresser against the wall. We keep all our delivery supplies in the closet and in the dresser, purposely out of sight of the laboring woman. The sight of oxygen tanks, needles, and scissors can make even the most relaxed woman feel tense. These things are taken out later if they're needed.

While Claire changed into a comfortable oversized T-shirt she'd brought from home, her husband went downstairs to the kitchen to get them both some lunch. We advise women to eat or drink during labor if they feel they want to. Most women in labor, however, prefer not to eat much. Claire was no exception— she opted for some fruit juice while Matthew had a sandwich. (Fathers rarely lose *their* appetites!)

At 2:00 P.M. contractions were still irregular but the baby's heart tones sounded fine. Claire was still only four centimeters dilated, but I could feel that the amniotic sac was bulging through the cervix, meaning that the baby's head wasn't resting directly against the cervix. I suggested that I rupture the membranes to try to speed things up. Claire was in enough labor to keep her from resting but not enough to make progress. When the membranes are ruptured and the amniotic fluid escapes from the uterus, the uterus gets a bit smaller and contracts more efficiently. The baby's head also pushes directly against the cervix and causes it to dilate faster. At this point, the woman will usually be moved into active labor. Claire agreed. I called in another nurse-midwife and she listened to the baby's heartbeat while I ruptured the membranes using a long plastic instrument that looks like a knitting needle. It looks awful, but it's really quite simple and painless! The fluid was clear, the baby's heartbeat good, and Claire moved into very productive labor.

The atmosphere in the room immediately changed. Claire and Matthew went from relaxed, joking old pros to an intense, serious laboring couple. Claire was standing up for much of the time, with her arms around Matthew's neck and shoulders, leaning into him with each contraction. Her face was flushed and she wasn't talking during contractions anymore. She started to perspire. Between contractions, she would still smile and listen to some small talk. I could see she was trying not to let the labor overwhelm her even though the contractions were very intense. I stayed with them for moral support and didn't leave the room. I rubbed her back and talked to her about relaxing and opening up during the contractions. In between contractions, I joked with her. I told her that labor was proof that God was a man because no woman would ever invent this! She laughed. Laughter is great during labor. It relaxes everyone. Things started to move very quickly now. Claire had delivered her last baby in under five hours and

I could see she was having another fast labor now. The contractions were right on top of one another and she began to shake. The body often shivers in response to labor. I kept telling her how well she was doing, and she would open her eyes and give me a quick smile for a few seconds.

In the middle of a big contraction, Claire caught her breath, gave a reflexive grunt, and with absolute certainty announced, "I've got to push." I always believe an experienced mother when she says this! If you ignore this voice, you will miss a lot of deliveries.

The baby had dropped down but the face was to the front instead of to the back. This position, called occiput posterior, or OP, makes it more difficult for the mother to push the baby down and out. Claire's other two babies had presented the same way, so this was no surprise for her, unfortunately. Pushing was hard. We had Claire try a number of positions (squatting, sitting, lying on her side) in an attempt to help her move this baby down and out. She was having intense lower back pain, so Jan (the other midwife), Matthew, and I did our best to make her comfortable. We put cold washcloths on her forehead, hot compresses on her perineum, and massaged her lower back. We gave her sips of juice after each contraction and told her she was making great progress, that she was almost there. At times she looked doubtful, but she kept working. After thirty minutes of pushing, the head crowned and in less than a minute the rest of the baby followed— a pink, healthy, slippery baby girl.

Matthew got soaked with the remaining amniotic fluid that flew out with the baby. He jumped off the bed and began to rummage around in his suitcase for what I assumed would be a dry pair of pants, but instead he pulled out a camera and began to take pictures of his crying wife and daughter. Claire was laughing and crying at the same time, thanking everyone. "I didn't think I could do it. Oh, you guys . . . this is great! Thanks!"

They were so thrilled to have a little girl. In these first few hours after a birth, I love my job the most. Claire nursed the baby while Matthew dialed the boys at home to tell them the news. It was peaceful and quiet, a time for Claire and Matthew to simply get to know their new child.

After an hour, the baby was weighed and measured and given a complete physical. Claire showered and ate a casserole that she and Matthew had brought from home (he heated it up in the microwave downstairs). Just four hours after the delivery, they left the birth center for home.

Two days later I visited them all at their home. The pediatrician had been there the day before and found the baby to be doing very well. When I arrived, Claire's mother was making dinner, Matthew was on the phone taking a business call, and Claire was reading to the boys from her bed while the baby slept in a friend's arms. The children knew me from the office visits and began to race around, showing me their toys, but they stopped to watch me check the baby over. Then they took turns taking pictures of me holding the baby.

Birth Center

A free-standing birth center is a facility separate, both physically and administratively, from a hospital. Most birth centers are operated by certified nurse-midwives or by physicians. These centers provide prenatal care, a site for labor and delivery, and postnatal care as well as well-woman gynecology. They were started to give women an alternative to hospital and home births. Birth centers are the ideal way for many women to have their babies in safety, peace, and quiet. For the low-risk mother and her baby, they often represent a good compromise between the intimacy of a home birth and the safety of a hospital birth.

Free-standing birth centers may be next door to a hospital, a few blocks away, or many miles away. They are always within easy reach of a hospital by ambulance. Emergency medical equipment—from oxygen to Isolettes—is also on hand at the center.

The birth center I helped to found in 1982 was modeled after my own home-birth practice. I knew how to do safe home births

and I knew what made them special. I felt that we could trans-
late all this knowledge and experience into a wonderful place
to have babies. We at the Maternity Center run a cheerful and
homelike facility that allows our staff of nurse-midwives to care
for every aspect of a woman's pregnancy, from prenatal checkups
through labor and delivery management plus postpartum follow-
ups. Our center, the Maternity Center Associates in Bethesda,
Maryland, is now the model for many others like it across the
country. Students are sent to our birth center to observe and
learn.

Women who wish to use a birth center like ours are carefully
screened to determine their low-risk status. Women with heart
disease, diabetes, or other serious health problems should not
deliver outside a hospital. Nor should women pregnant with multiple fetuses. Any serious problem that should unexpectedly arise
during the course of prenatal care would be referred to a backup
physician working in consultation with the birth-center staff.
Emergencies that occur during labor, delivery, or postpartum
would be transferred immediately to waiting backup physicians
at the hospital.

It's easy for me to find satisfaction in my work at the birth
center because the mothers and fathers who deliver there are so
happy with the experience. They appreciate being able to give
birth in the warm, familiar atmosphere of the birth center instead
of in a busy, unfamiliar hospital. Those who have given birth
previously in hospitals have told me after a birth-center birth that
they are convinced that normal healthy mothers and babies do
not belong in the hospital atmosphere.

ADVANTAGES OF A BIRTH CENTER

1. A birth center provides individualized care in a nonthreatening
   setting.
2. Pregnancy is considered a natural and healthy process.
3. During prenatal care, women are encouraged to take charge
   of their own health care. For example, patients at the Maternity Center are encouraged to read and understand all that

is written about them and to participate in decision-making. If they don't understand the medical jargon or any notations made about them, we want them to ask us to explain it. Women especially like reviewing their medical chart of a past pregnancy; they are fascinated by the formerly mysterious medical record that tells *their* delivery story. Each woman learns how to test her own urine and record the results on her chart. She also weighs herself and records the figure.

4. Patients are encouraged to bring family members (children, grandparents, husbands) with them to the prenatal visits. Often grandmothers-to-be ask as many questions as their daughters and are thrilled to hear the baby's heartbeat through the Doppler. Children who frequently accompany their mothers get used to the routine and enjoy the homey atmosphere, like the three-year-old who said, "Go lie down, Mommy, we gots to measure you and listen to the baby."

5. During the birth, family members and friends are allowed at the parents' discretion. Children may be at the center for the birth and may come in to see the delivery as well.

6. Birth centers are small; they are not large, impersonal bureaucracies like some hospitals.

7. Rules, restrictions, and policies are few and flexible.

8. Mothers may go home soon after delivery. After birth, mothers and babies are discharged from the center within eight hours. Careful follow-up care is given by the staff through phone calls, home visits, and center visits. The baby is checked out by the center's staff right after delivery, and a pediatrician sees the newborn within forty-eight hours of delivery.

DISADVANTAGES OF A BIRTH CENTER

1. You may have to be moved to a hospital during labor if there are warning signs of maternal or fetal distress. This possibility must be taken into consideration when deciding on a birth center. (At the Maternity Center, only about 10 percent of our laboring mothers need to be transferred to the hospital. Less than 1 percent need to go by ambulance.)

2. The facilities for serious emergencies are not on-site; they are an ambulance ride away.
3. You cannot stay for a two- or three-day rest. You will be discharged from a birth center within four to twenty-four hours.
4. There are no on-site pediatricians and no nursery for the baby.
5. You may find that you are not able to deliver at a birth center due to your medical history. Birth centers can accept only low-risk mothers.

Questions to Ask About Birth Centers

The birth center you choose should work within a system that provides for problems and emergencies. The health-care professionals at the center must be highly skilled in maternity care.

Some questions you may want to ask at the birth center when you tour:

How do you determine which women can safely deliver here? What types of deliveries cannot be done here? Why?
The midwives at a birth center should screen you to determine if you are a high- or low-risk patient. They should ask you questions about serious illnesses such as diabetes, any past pregnancies and their outcomes, and personal habits such as smoking and drinking. Women with breech babies, premature babies, multiple fetuses, pregnancy-induced hypertension (PIH), or preexisting diabetes are not good candidates for a birth center.

What provisions do you have for emergencies at deliveries?
Most centers will have the ability to resuscitate the infant, IV equipment, certain drugs to stop postpartum hemorrhage, a Doppler to listen to fetal heart tones, oxygen, and a good transport system in case you have to be moved to the hospital.

Which drugs cannot be used at the center?
Pitocin to speed labor is not usually used at a birth center, nor are most painkillers.

Who is your backup physician? What hospital is he or she affiliated with?
You may want to meet this person just in case he or she has to help out during your birth.

Who manages the labor and delivery? The midwife on call or the same midwife who handles my prenatal care?
It is important to find out how the group works. Most groups have an "on call" system, and your baby will be delivered by the CNM on duty at the time. This ensures that you have a rested and alert midwife.

What happens immediately after birth? Who checks out the baby? Who administers eye drops? Injections? Is a heel-stick blood test done?
Usually both the midwife and later a pediatrician will check the baby. Ask if you need to contact a pediatrician in advance.

What is the philosophy of the center?
Try to get an idea of how a normal labor and delivery are handled.

How long has the center been in existence?
You may feel more comfortable with one that has a long history and good reputation.

What do the outcome statistics look like? How many women are transferred to a hospital during labor? How many of these women end up needing a cesarean or forceps delivery? How many women hemorrhage? What is the rate of infant or maternal deaths? Were any babies born with brain damage?
All these statistics will give a good indication of how well the center screens pregnant women for high-risk problems and how good it is at handling normal labor and birth. You should not find that large numbers of women are being moved to the hospital during labor.

How far is the center from the hospital?
The center should place you no farther than thirty minutes from a hospital delivery table equipped for a C-section. Do not count door-to-door time. Count door-to-operating-table time.

What is the most common reason for a move to the hospital?
At our center, failure to progress in labor is the most common reason for a transfer. Failure to progress in labor does not indicate any present danger to the fetus, nor does it necessarily mean a cesarean will be required. Indeed, it rarely signifies a true, time-is-of-the-essence emergency. The woman is moved so that the labor, which is not progressing by nondrug means, can be made productive with Pitocin. Pitocin can cause fetal distress and most birth centers do not use it during labor. If the center is next door to the hospital, however, it may be able to administer Pitocin. If the woman is not transferred and given Pitocin, she will eventually become exhausted and, if she is left long enough, there may be fetal distress.

Do the midwives at the center also have hospital privileges?
In the event of an emergency move to the hospital you'll want to know if your midwife will be able to accompany you there and stay with you. Although it's nice if the midwife has hospital privileges and can actually deliver babies at the hospital, this is not always the case. The CNM should at least stay with you to help establish a plan of care and to support you emotionally.

Are the midwives at the center certified nurse-midwives? Who assists the nurse-midwife at the birth, another CNM or a nurse?
The center should be run by licensed certified nurse-midwives. Someone should always assist at the birth—either another CNM or a labor-and-delivery nurse.

Is the center licensed? Is it accredited by the National Association of Childbearing Centers?
Make sure that it is. If it has been accredited by the NACC, it has passed the rigorous standards set by this organization. See address on the next page.

What is the birth center's view on episiotomies? How often are they done?
If you hope to avoid an episiotomy, you'll want to choose a birth center that shares your view.

Who can be with the mother during labor/delivery?
Almost any birth center will allow the father or support person

to be with you, but if you want children and other relatives or friends, it's always wise to ask about the center's policy. There may, for example, be commonsense restrictions on the number of people attending the birth.

How soon after delivery do most women go home?
Usually women leave birth centers within four to twenty-four hours after delivery. Find out what the norm is at your center. Do not expect a hospital-like stay of three days, complete with food service!

Check the list of questions at the end of the hospital section, on pages 47–51. Many of these hospital-related queries may also be appropriate to ask at a birth center. For further information on birth centers, write or call the National Association of Child-bearing Centers, Route 1, Box 1, Perkiomenville, PA 18075 (215–234–8068). For a list of birth centers near you, enclose one dollar to cover postage and handling.

The Hospital Experience

Cathy chose to have her first baby at a hospital because it felt "safer" to her. She knew she would be just down the hall from operating rooms, anesthesiologists, and an intensive-care nursery. She chose a major city hospital, a tertiary-care facility, which means it is equipped to handle seriously ill patients and critically sick babies. The hospital's intensive-care nursery is a model for the best neonatology has to offer. Even though she had no reason to think she would need this kind of help, Cathy felt better knowing it was there for her and her baby.

It was 11:00 P.M. when I walked into the lobby of this six-story hospital spreading across two city blocks. The lobby is usually bustling with doctors, visitors, patients, social workers, and nurses, but at this time of night the hallways were quiet. The gift shop was darkened and locked. A sole guard sat at the front desk. My shoes echoed as I walked down the black-and-white-tiled halls to the elevator in the east wing. Even the elevator was waiting and empty. Night deliveries have that advantage. Parents can usually make it all the way to labor and delivery without having to deal with the hubbub typical of hospitals during the day. I got in and pushed 5, for the "L&D" floor.

As soon as the doors opened, I saw Cathy and Scott standing at the nurses' station filling out a number of hospital forms. In order to be admitted, the nurse needed to get the patient's medical history and some consent forms signed about circumcision, C-sections, and infant care. Then she showed them down the hall to the birthing room. Cathy had requested the birthing room (for low-risk mothers), and luckily it was empty so we could use it. The hospital has only one birthing room—a large room with private bath attached. It was like the rest of the L&D suite, windowless. Its new decor and wood furniture made it look less like a hospital and more like a motel room. Most of the doctors delivering patients in this hospital feel more comfortable using the delivery rooms, so the birthing room is almost always free. The birthing room is located at the end of a long hall, across from the delivery rooms. The advantage to this location is that it is removed from the general commotion of the floor and there is little traffic. Few uninvited guests (nurses, medical students, residents) are likely to wander in to watch the birth. The disadvantage: if I needed someone in a hurry, I couldn't just open the door and yell. I would have to use the intercom, speak to the nurse manning the front desk, and get her to send help, hoping she would get the message that it was urgent!

Sally, the nurse on duty, helped Cathy change into a hospital gown that tied up the back. She took Cathy's street clothes and put them in a plastic bag with her name on it. I meanwhile went to get into the obligatory hospital scrubs. The first thing I did when I came into the birthing room was to check the delivery supplies and emergency supplies to make sure everything was in the room. Since the birthing room was still not used regularly at this hospital, the staff sometimes forgot to restock it. I know a lot of people worry about supplies being on hand at a home birth or birth center, but in my practice I had my biggest worries about supplies when I used the hospital birthing room.

To complete Cathy's admission process, the hospital also required some blood work and an admission physical to assess the mother's general health, the status of her labor, and, of course, the fetal heartbeat. We'd worked out an agreement with the hospital that, unless there was a problem, we would use the fetal monitor only intermittently instead of strapping it on for the whole labor.

Cathy was four centimeters dilated, the beginning of serious labor. At this point, for some women, the labor begins to hurt and may start to feel overwhelming. Cathy was coping by walking around, between the birthing room and the adjoining bathroom. We were discouraged from letting our patients walk in the hallways. The labor floor is a busy place and privacy is difficult to maintain. A walk past the four delivery rooms and six labor rooms would provide the unsuspecting newcomer with views of half-covered women in varying stages of labor and birth.

Cathy began to walk faster and faster between contractions. She tried the shower, she tried sitting on the toilet, then on the bed, then in a chair. She looked like she was trying to run away from the labor, and seemed to be trying to hold back this powerful, scary force. She said she was trying to find "the right position," which for her meant a place where the contractions wouldn't hurt. I rubbed Cathy's back, and Scott tried to get her to relax by breathing with her as they had practiced in prenatal classes. But Cathy only grew more tense and anxious.

Picking up on this, I talked to her as honestly and plainly as I could. "You need to face some facts about this labor. It's going to get a lot stronger before this baby can come out. You can't dance around anymore to avoid it. We are all right here to help you because it is tough and it can be scary, but *you* have to do this. No one can do it for you. You need to let go and let this labor happen. I know you can do it."

She looked at me soberly and said, "Okay, I will." And she did! In two hours, she was eight centimeters dilated, working really hard and concentrating on relaxing. It's not easy to give in to nature and go with the flow, but this is the key to successful labor.

Just then a nurse stuck her head in and motioned for me to come into the hall (always an ominous sign!). Apparently, some of the obstetricians down the hall were grumbling. They wanted to know where my backup doctor was. According to hospital policy, the backup obstetrician had to be on the floor during the delivery (even if he was asleep in the lounge!). I thanked her for letting me know and assured the nurse that he was on his way and would arrive on time.

"Anything wrong?" asked Cathy and Scott when I walked back in. "No," I lied. "They just wanted to know what I want on my pizza—they're ordering out." Hospital politics and grumblings are the last thing a woman in labor needs to hear about! I feel it's my job to keep out the negative vibes and let the parents-to-be concentrate on themselves.

My backup OB arrived and came in for a quick hello. He told Cathy, "Looks great; it won't be long now." Then he retired to the lounge to watch TV and wait. Within the hour, Cathy was fully dilated (at ten centimeters) and ready to push. We adjusted the bed and the pillows so that Cathy could be in a semisitting position for the birth. After one and a half hours of sweaty push-ing, lots of coaching, ice chips, and encouragement, out came baby Joshua, kicking and screaming. I lifted him onto his moth-er's chest and the nurse covered them both with warm blankets. Scott and Cathy greeted the baby with exhausted joy and great enthusiasm. Cathy thanked us for all the support and help and kept repeating, "I don't believe this; he's really here! I couldn't have done it without you." The truth was, I couldn't have done it without *her*!

For the moment, the nurse held back on all the hospital rou-tines for immediate baby care (footprints, eye drops, etc.) and let the family get acquainted. I showed Cathy how to nurse the baby while he was awake and alert. Joshua obligingly opened his eyes, which amazed and delighted his parents. Like most new parents, they immediately realized he was the most wonderful baby in the world.

Cathy checked into a hospital room for her two-day stay. The baby was placed in a bassinet beside her and Scott went home to get some rest before returning the next morning. I finished up my paperwork and then drove home in the early morning light, humming and smiling to myself.

I must say that the hospital birth described above is, unfortunately, not always the norm. As a midwife delivering there, I attempted to allow the mother to give birth without a lot of intervention. Most hospital births, however, are actively and rigidly managed according to hospital policy and traditions. This often means that the mother ends up having IVs, fetal monitors, painkillers, and other medical interventions, even if they're not really *necessary*. Often one intervention leads to another, and normal labor and delivery can become complicated. At the risk of being called antihospital (which I'm not), a *typical* hospital labor and delivery might go more like this:

A woman goes into labor and phones her doctor. He or she tells her to go to the hospital to be checked.

On arrival at the hospital, she is given a vaginal exam by an OB resident, or nurse, whom she has never met before. Her doctor is not there yet.

The nurse hooks her up to an IV; she tells her that IVs are always used (in case she bleeds or needs an emergency C-section, it's already in place). Then she hooks her up to a fetal monitor, telling her that continuous electronic fetal monitoring is the safest thing for the baby. Because of these two procedures, the woman is now basically confined to bed. The nurse may also give an enema, based on doctor's orders, to empty the lower bowel and speed up the labor.

Medical and obstetrical history is taken down and consent forms are signed.

The nurse leaves the room; the mother and coach remain alone to cope with labor. They can busy themselves by staring at the fetal monitor and a big clock on the wall. She is only four centimeters dilated so the doctor hasn't come yet. (The nurse is keeping him apprised of all activity by phone.)

At five centimeters, the doctor arrives and does another vaginal exam. He ruptures the membranes and attaches an internal monitor to get a better indication of fetal health. Now the woman is definitely confined to bed (she can't get up because of the internal fetal monitor). When she has to urinate, she is offered a bedpan.

At six centimeters the woman complains about the pain of labor. The doctor says, "Well, you've got a long way to go yet," but suggests that she "hold out a little longer" before taking anything.

At seven centimeters she complains some more and so he suggests an epidural. He says epidurals are very popular because they don't depress the baby's breathing and the mother stays awake and feels no pain. He does not tell her much about the possible side effects of the drug (the package insert required by the U.S. Food and Drug Administration contains a long list of unwanted side effects).

She takes the epidural and feels much better (though strange, since she's numb from the waist down). Unfortunately, the relaxing effect of the epidural relaxes the labor too, and contractions are slowing down. (This is one of those side effects that is often not mentioned.)

Because labor has slowed down considerably, the doctor suggests Pitocin, a synthetic hormone that works to contract the uterus and will speed things up.

Labor speeds up but the contractions are hard on the baby. The baby's heart rate begins to dip with each contraction and he is showing signs of fetal distress (due to the Pitocin the mother has been given). The woman is given oxygen and turned on her side in an effort to reduce stress to the baby.

Luckily, she is now fully dilated and begins to push, but, due to the epidural, she doesn't really feel the urge to push. (Women with epidurals frequently lose the power to push well.) She is moved to the delivery room because forceps must now be used to help her get the baby out. The doctor does an episiotomy and uses outlet forceps to deliver the baby.

The delivery room is cold so the baby gets cold and is whisked off to the nursery to get warm.

The mother can't go to the nursery because the epidural hasn't worn off yet, so she waits in her room. Four to eight hours later, she is brought her baby and she holds him for the first time.

A similar scenario might just as easily have ended with a cesarean. The startling facts today are that one in every four women entering the hospital to give birth will deliver surgically—by cesarean. In some areas this statistic soars even higher (around 30 percent of the births in my area of the country are now by C-section). I don't mean to condemn the use of forceps, epidurals, and C-sections for all women in all circumstances, but I do feel they are overused by many doctors in hospital settings.

The Hospital

Hospitals are classified three ways: primary care, secondary care, and tertiary care. A primary-care center is appropriate for low-risk births. At a primary-care center there is often no anesthesiologist on the floor and so at least thirty minutes are needed to set up for a C-section. A secondary-care hospital can handle moderate-risk deliveries. A tertiary-care facility can handle high-risk births and babies. They have intensive-care nurseries for premature and critically ill babies. Secondary- and tertiary-care hospitals can usually do emergency C-sections immediately (within five to ten minutes).

Most women in the United States currently feel safer in a hospital and so choose to deliver there. Others choose the hospital simply because other options (home, birth center) are not considered or don't exist in their areas.

Hospital births, although currently the most common, are a relatively new concept in the historical span of things. Not until the 1950s did hospitals dominate the scene. Before 1900 hospital births were highly unusual. Only the very sick were brought in to deliver there. By the 1940s about half of the births were taking place in hospitals, but by 1970, over 99 percent of births were performed in hospitals, usually by male physicians. With early hospital births (before 1950) came the use of anesthesia for childbirth and separation of the baby from the mother and the mother from the family. Hospitals have changed over the years to meet consumer demand for more flexible, family-oriented births. Happily, hospitals are still changing to suit the needs and demands of today's laboring mother.

Hospitals, because they vary so much in size, type, and policy, can be hard to assess as a group. Hospitals can run the spectrum from the very traditional to the very flexible. Most hospitals are somewhere in between. You will want to arrange a tour of the hospital so you can see for yourself what this hospital is all about. It will also give you the chance to ask questions about hospital policy as it relates to childbirth and newborn care. Find out who gives the tour. Is it a labor-and-delivery nurse? A childbirth educator? At the hospital where I used to practice, the nurses took turns leading tours. Some made the place sound wonderful; others could make it sound like a jail! Keep in mind that the person who leads your tour probably has strong feelings about the place where she works.

Although hospital policy is very important, the way your practitioner works within these policies is even more so. Some may bend and stretch strict hospital rules to fit their own style, while others may never take advantage of flexible hospital policies. The hospital you tour may have nicely decorated birthing rooms, labor rooms with bath attached, birthing chairs, rooming-in policies, and the like. But when asked how often these facilities are used, you may find that the answer is "rarely." In fact, most mothers delivering in hospitals still end up on the delivery table with anesthesia. The birthing room may be no more than window dressing set up to meet consumer demand for a more homey setting. Some birthing rooms are not even decorated but look just like delivery rooms. The only difference: a birthing bed instead of a delivery table and the benefit of not having to move from labor room to delivery room during labor. After birth in a hospital, babies are often routinely separated from their mothers for up to twelve hours and "rooming-in" may in practice mean only between nine and twelve noon or two and six P.M. It is important to dig beneath the surface and find out not only what is *allowed* but what is *encouraged*. It is far better to be in a hospital that *routinely* runs the way you would like it to than to have to fight the system.

To cut through the glossy exterior and find out what really goes on in the hospital, ask how many people use the birthing rooms, what percentage of the mothers choose to breast-feed, how many people room in with their newborns, whether the baby must spend any time in the nursery (such as during visiting hours or at night). This will help you to assess whether hospital "policies" really represent hospital "practices." (See the section on page 47 on questions to ask.)

If while touring a hospital and asking questions you discover certain statistics that aren't in keeping with your wishes (for example, if you hope to avoid anesthesia but find that only 15 percent of women at this hospital do avoid it), think long and hard about this. Do not fool yourself into assuming you will be one of the 15 percent that breeze through labor without a pain-killer. The numbers are not in your favor. They indicate an atmosphere in which women are encouraged to rely on drugs for birth.

ADVANTAGES OF A HOSPITAL BIRTH

1. If you plan to give birth at a high-risk hospital, the benefit is that no matter what happens, you won't have to change your plans. Everything you could need for yourself or your baby would be available right there. High-risk centers are best at handling serious problems such as prematurity, life-threatening birth defects, neonatal surgery, multiple births, and mothers with diabetes or other serious diseases. This does not mean, however, that a hospital can ensure absolute safety

or a foolproof remedy for every crisis. It just means that the facilities and staff are *there*.

2. Hospitals are the only facilities that can do cesareans. A C-section cannot be performed at home or in a birth center. An *emergency* C-section is done when the baby's heart-rate pattern shows signs of severe distress, indicating that the baby is no longer receiving adequate oxygen. Usually, severe fetal distress is preceded by mild to moderate fetal distress.

3. Hospitals are also the best places to be if you feel safest there. Each woman needs to honestly evaluate her own feelings about birth. If she only feels safe delivering in a hospital, that is where she belongs. In order for women to relax in labor they need to feel safe and secure. I once had a woman attempt to deliver at the Maternity Center, but she was not progressing in labor. As time went on it became clearer and clearer that, although she had talked herself into the birth center, she would feel secure only in a hospital setting. I moved her to the hospital and, sure enough, labor immediately picked up and her baby was born soon after without incident.

4. The mother who stays in the hospital for a few days after delivery ideally has round-the-clock help for herself and her baby from the medical and nursing staff. In a well-run hospital she should have plenty of time to learn about feeding, ask questions, be shown how to give the baby a bath, etc. If she decides she wants a rest, she can send the baby to the nursery to be cared for there.

5. An on-staff pediatrician or neonatologist will examine your baby within the first twelve to twenty-four hours. You do not have to take the baby anywhere or arrange to have a pediatrician come to your home.

6. If your baby has any special needs or medical problems, intermediate or intensive care is often available. (At many hospitals, however, particularly primary- and secondary-care ones, a very sick baby has to be moved to another hospital with better nursery facilities.)

DISADVANTAGES OF A HOSPITAL BIRTH

1. Hospitals may make you feel like a sick person.
2. Hospitals often seem cold, impersonal, and intimidating.
3. Patients in the hospital face a 25 to 30 percent chance of C-section.
4. There is a greater chance of unnecessary medical intervention during a hospital delivery.
5. You have a lack of privacy. Unknown doctors, residents, fellows, and nurses tend to wander in and out, sometimes talking about you as though you aren't even there.
6. As large institutions, hospitals must have policies and rules and red tape. They rarely bend to accommodate the individual.
7. One disadvantage of a high-risk center, if you happen to have a normal birth, is that your labor is being managed by experts trained in pathology (the study of the abnormal). They know how to manage serious birthing difficulties but may have little or no experience with normal unmedicated births. As such, your birth may be unnecessarily interfered with, because the use of modern technical interventions is the norm here.
8. At all hospitals, there is a good chance that your baby will spend time in the nursery, away from you.
9. Hospitals are often noisy, making it difficult for new mothers to sleep.
10. Rules regarding visitors are often restrictive and inflexible. The baby may be sent to the nursery during visiting hours, meaning that grandparents, siblings, and friends are unable to hold or be with the baby.

Questions to Ask About Hospital Births

Here are some other questions you may want to get answered about the hospital you tour:

Who can be with me in labor? How many coaches/people can be in the room with me? May the coach remain in the event of a cesarean?
A support person provides you with the emotional support you need. You'll want to know if there are any restrictions on that person's presence.

Are children allowed to visit during labor? Can they be present at the birth? Who will take care of them?
Not all hospitals allow children at the birth. If they do, find out if you should bring a baby-sitter.

Is there a mandatory enema or shave on admission?
Remember, even if your doctor says it's not mandatory but the hospital routinely does it, you may end up with an admitting nurse or resident who, in your doctor's absence, pushes for standard hospital procedure.

During vaginal exams and other procedures does the coach have to leave the room? What is the thinking behind this?
In many hospitals, the coach is routinely asked to step out to the hall during vaginal exams, leaving the mother without her support person.

Is there a preadmission form that can be filled out to avoid hassles on admission? Who first examines me? A labor nurse? A resident? Or does my obstetrician or midwife usually arrive in time to ensure continuity of care?
If you can, fill out preadmission forms to avoid bureaucratic entanglements at check-in. If you prefer to be examined only by your CNM or doctor, see if you can avoid having a nurse or resident examine you on arrival.

Will I be allowed or encouraged to walk around during labor? What if my water has already broken?
Walking can help the labor progress. Many hospitals do not allow it. In some hospitals, once the membranes have broken, the woman is confined to bed. But as long as the heart rate indicates that the baby is fine, it is safe to walk around and there is no real reason to be confined to bed. Try to find a hospital that runs according to your needs and wishes.

Can I eat during labor? Drink soft drinks? Tea? Have ice chips?
Find out what is allowed and bring it with you to the hospital.
Don't depend on having tea or ice cubes waiting for you.

Are IVs routine? Do most doctors or midwives order them?
You may want to try to avoid an IV. See pages 171–172.

Is continuous electronic fetal monitoring standard? Are there exceptions?
If not continuous, does the fetal monitor have to be used for a minimum
number of times during the labor?
Again, this is a routine you may wish to avoid. If so, you'll want
to find a hospital that does not insist on continuous monitoring.
For more on this, see pages 181–183.

Where are the bathrooms? Or are bedpans the rule?
You'll probably feel more comfortable if you have use of a bathroom.

Is each woman assigned a nurse? How many patients does one nurse
have to watch at one time?
One nurse should not have to care for more than two laboring
women at the same time.

How many deliveries are there on an average day?
Try to find out whether the hospital facilities and staff are over-
worked.

How many birthing rooms/delivery rooms are there? What percentage
of women actually use the birthing room? What percentage use the delivery
rooms?
If you hope to use the birthing room, you'll want to know whether
it's likely to happen. Some hospitals have birthing rooms but
don't seem comfortable using them.

Are labor rooms shared with other laboring patients?
Some hospitals have more than one bed in a labor room, and it
may make you uncomfortable to have "company" during your
labor. Also, some hospitals first put laboring mothers into a
multiple-bed admitting room. Find out about this.

Do most women delivering here use a table and stirrups for delivery?
Can I deliver on my side or squatting if that works better for me?
For the happiest match, try to find a hospital that fits your philosophy of birth.

Are episiotomies routinely done here? Are there any MDs on staff who don't routinely do them?
If they're done as a matter of course, they may be hard to avoid. See pages 166–171 for more on avoiding episiotomies.

Are there anesthesiologists in the hospital twenty-four hours a day? Are they on call at home?
At some hospitals at night and on weekends, the anesthesiologist is on call and it may take about twenty minutes to get him or her there, as much as another twenty to set up for the C-section. So in reality it takes as long to set up some hospitals for C-sections as it does to transfer a woman from a birth center to a hospital for a C-section.

Are there residents in obstetrics in the hospital?
On the positive side, residents mean that if you get to the hospital and need to deliver before your physician gets there, an experienced doctor will be on hand to deliver the baby. On the negative side, however, you may be left in the hands of this resident by a doctor who depends on him or her to manage the labor. Some doctors prefer to arrive in time only for the actual delivery. This means that the caregiver you have communicated your wishes to isn't there to make sure your labor is conducted according to those wishes.

Do nurse-midwives have privileges at the hospital? Do they do deliveries or work as nurses?
Often hospitals with CNMs are a little more flexible/liberal than ones who have no CNMs on staff.

What is the routine immediately after birth? Do healthy babies go to the nursery to be bathed/weighed/checked or do they usually stay with their parents?
If you want to keep your baby with you, make sure the hospital rules allow this.

Is there an early-discharge program for healthy babies and mothers? How many hours after birth can they be discharged?
Many women prefer to go home and sleep in their own beds. Find out who would check the baby and mothers for problems after an early discharge. Some hospitals send out RNs to make house calls on day two and day three. They check for jaundice and help with breast-feeding problems.

What is the policy on rooming in with the baby? Are there any hours when the baby is taken to the nursery?
If you want twenty-four-hour rooming-in, make sure that the hospital rules allow this.

Is breast-feeding encouraged? Does the baby routinely get bottles of water or formula? What about feeding problems? Is there special help for breast-feeding mothers? Is there a milk bank (where mothers' pumped breast milk is stored for later use) at the hospital?
A milk bank may be a good sign that knowledgeable people are there.

Are the neonatologists in the hospital twenty-four hours a day? Are they available for consultation?
If the hospital does not have a neonatal intensive-care unit, you'll want to know where babies go if the hospital cannot care for them.

How many babies are treated for jaundice?
Normal physiological jaundice is present in about 30 percent of all normal newborns but needs treatment in only a small percentage of cases. The need for treatment is determined by the bilirubin levels in the newborn's blood.

What are the visiting hours? May children visit? May children hold the baby? May someone spend the night if I have a private room? Are there special telephoning hours?
Some hospitals have a long list of rules regarding visiting; they may not even take incoming calls for you after a certain hour at night. Their policies may affect your choice of hospital.

Now that you have chosen your caregiver and a location for the birth, you'll want to turn your thoughts inward. The coming chapters will give you information on prenatal care, advice on good nutrition, and ways to cope with the changes and discomforts of pregnancy.

3

Prenatal Care

Once you have chosen a midwife or doctor, you will begin to see him or her monthly during your pregnancy. The purpose of these visits is to monitor your health and your baby's growth. Your caregiver will also remain on the lookout for serious pregnancy-related conditions that may affect you or your baby and that need prompt medical attention. In this chapter we will cover fetal development, prenatal checkups, and some of the medical problems that may come up during your pregnancy.

How Does Your Baby Grow?

You may be wondering just what is happening inside you. How is your baby developing? If you could peek inside, this is what you'd see:

5 weeks: Your baby's heart begins to beat, although the sound cannot yet be picked up by a Doppler. Brain, spinal cord, arms and legs, eyes, nose, and mouth begin to develop. Your baby is about one-quarter inch long.

8 weeks: Your baby is making tiny movements, but you cannot

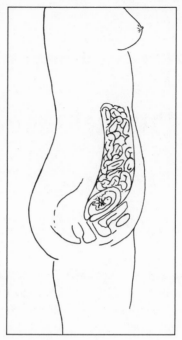

Nine weeks

feel them yet. Your baby's face is forming. The embryo is now 1⅛ inches long.

10 weeks: Your baby's eyes are closed. Testes or ovaries have formed.

11 weeks: Your baby's movements become more vigorous, but you still can't feel the kicking yet.

12 weeks: Your baby makes breathing and swallowing motions. Your baby weighs only an ounce. The heartbeat is audible with a Doppler (ultrasound stethoscope) at your doctor's or CNM's office.

16 weeks: Your baby has developed a sense of taste. He or she may get the hiccups. If a bright light were shone on your abdomen, your baby's heart rate would speed up and he or she

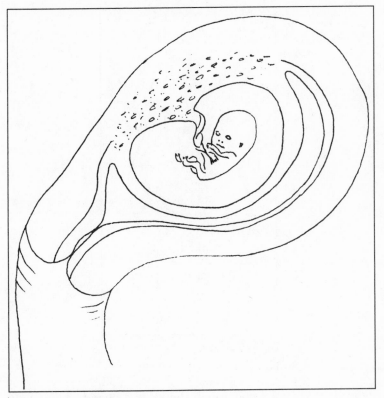

Actual size of the fetus at nine weeks

would turn his or her head away. Downy hair, known as lanugo, covers the body, which is now six to eight inches long and weighs four to six ounces.

18 weeks: Your baby's movements might now be felt by you. Toenails are developing.

20 weeks: Your baby's heartbeat is now audible with a regular unamplified fetoscope. Your baby may suck his or her thumb.

21 weeks: Your baby can make a fist. Your baby's skin is red and wrinkled.

22 weeks: Your baby begins to make more definite sucking motions.

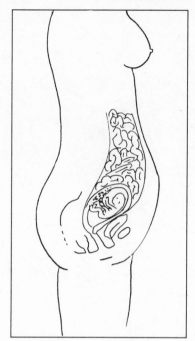

Eighteen weeks

24 weeks: Your baby now weighs between a pound and a pound and a half.

26 weeks: Your baby may move about when it hears loud noises. Your baby has eyelashes. The body is still very thin.

27 weeks: Your baby makes stronger breathing motions now. The baby won't breathe air until birth, but begins to practice early in fetal life.

28 weeks: It is assumed that by this point the baby is "conscious," based on brain development. Your baby weighs about two to three pounds. Breathing is still a very rudimentary skill. Your baby can open his or her eyes.

32 weeks: Your baby experiences two types of sleep: REM (rapid-eye-movement sleep, in which adults dream), and non-REM

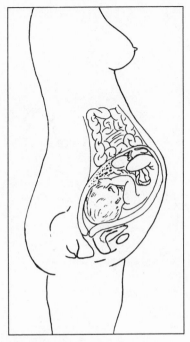

Twenty-six weeks

sleep, a deep, nondreaming state. Your baby weighs four or five pounds and is about seventeen or eighteen inches long.

34 weeks: Your baby responds to familiar voices.

36 weeks: The baby moves about once every ten minutes, but you won't be able to feel all of these movements. The skin is less wrinkled and the lanugo is almost gone. Your baby weighs about six pounds.

39 weeks: Your baby is asleep 95 percent of the time. Even in sleep, the baby moves and makes sucking motions.

40 weeks: At birth, your baby will weigh an average of seven pounds.

NOTE: The American College of Nurse-Midwives has a pregnancy wheel that includes information on growth and develop-

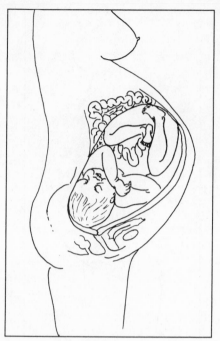

Forty weeks (full term)

ment. Send $2.50 to: ACNM, 1522 K Street, N.W., Suite 1000, Washington, D.C. 20005.

What Happens at Prenatal Checkups

What happens during prenatal checkups? Whether you've chosen a doctor or nurse-midwife, the same basic routine is followed. Appointments are scheduled monthly until the twenty-eighth week (seven months). You will then be seen every two weeks through the eighth month and weekly in your ninth. During these visits, your practitioner will get information on your health and your baby's. You will have the opportunity to ask questions, prepare for labor, and get to know your caretaker. Over the course of prenatal care, a relationship of respect, trust, and mutual understanding is ideally built. At each visit, your practitioner will:

1. Weigh you to monitor your gains.
2. Check your blood pressure to make sure it's normal.
3. Test your urine for protein and sugar. These tests indicate possible pregnancy-related illnesses such as toxemia and diabetes.
4. Measure your expanding abdomen from pubic bone to top of the uterus, or fundus. This gives valuable information on the growth rate of the fetus. The practitioner will also feel manually for the location and position of the baby. After twenty-eight weeks, an experienced hand can discern head from buttocks, arms, and legs.
5. Listen to the baby's heartbeat, using a Doppler or a fetascope. A Doppler is a hand-held ultrasound device that picks up fetal heart tones and amplifies them. Heart tones can be heard using this method by twelve weeks. A fetascope is a stethoscope with an adaptor that enables you to hear the heartbeat. It cannot amplify the sound. Fetal heart tones can be detected by about twenty weeks using a fetascope.

Routine Tests During Prenatal Visits

Internal exams are not normally done during pregnancy, with the exception of your first visit (for a Pap smear) and your final month's visits. Internals are done in between in case of vaginal infection or other problems.

A *blood sample* is taken early in pregnancy to determine your blood type, blood count, iron level, exposure to syphilis, and German measles. Sometimes, titers for toxoplasmosis, cytomegalovirus, and herpes are also drawn, especially if the mother is at risk for these diseases. They should ideally be done before the woman becomes pregnant, and repeated again during pregnancy if exposure to these viruses is suspected.

Urinalysis is done to check for bladder or kidney infections that may not produce symptoms.

Another blood test is done at sixteen to twenty-one weeks to determine the level of *alpha fetoprotein* (*AFP*) in the mother's blood. High levels may indicate spina bifida (a neural-tube defect). Low levels have been associated with a greater incidence of Down's syndrome. In either of these cases, a sonogram and amniocentesis would probably be recommended to determine whether or not a neural-tube defect or Down's syndrome actually exists. (See below.) Often, the original AFP test is misleading; this test has a high rate of false positives, meaning it often indicates a problem that does not in fact exist.

During the pregnancy, a *glucose test* is also done to determine the possibility of pregnancy-related diabetes. (A midwife usually will not independently handle the delivery of a woman with diabetes due to the high-risk nature of this pregnancy. This patient would be sent to an obstetrician or perinatologist or her care might be jointly managed by a CNM and an MD, depending on the severity of the disease.)

Although not routinely done during pregnancy, blood tests for AIDS are now available upon request for anyone wanting to know her AIDS status. A positive HIV (human immunovirus) means that you have been exposed to the AIDS virus. It does not mean you have the disease yet. The incubation period can be five to ten years. Mothers who carry the AIDS virus can pass it along to their unborn babies. Between thirty and fifty percent of babies of infected mothers will acquire AIDS.

Other Prenatal Tests

SONOGRAM

During a sonogram, the expectant mother lies on her back and a gel is spread on her abdomen. Then a metal instrument, a transducer, is moved over the abdomen. Sound waves are bounced off the fetus and depicted on a TV screen as an image. The test can help to determine the baby's due date, the amount of amniotic fluid, the presence of any gross physical abnormalities, the location and position of the baby, and any spinal cord defects. For the parents, a sonogram is usually joyous and exciting—an opportunity to see that there is a real baby in there. This can be an emotional lift, especially during the first trimester when you feel exhausted and nauseated with "nothing to show for it."

The safety of the sonogram has been studied extensively. Although there is currently no evidence that the sonogram is risky, there's no reason to perform one on everybody. This ultrasound procedure is certainly warranted in many cases but need not be done on all pregnant women. Repeated use of sonograms over the course of a low-risk pregnancy seems unjustified. The tests are expensive and there are no studies yet that show routine sonograms during normal pregnancy produce better outcomes for infants. Also, it is wise to be cautious about any relatively new technology for pregnancy. In the past we have seen other seemingly safe interventions become the cause of problems twenty or more years later.

If there are medical indications for concern (suspected twins, confusion over dates, possible ectopic pregnancy, or fibroids of the uterus), then the sonogram can give very valuable information. Sonogram technology is rapidly changing. Best results are achieved at a high-risk center with the latest equipment and the most experienced practitioner.

AMNIOCENTESIS

This test can be done for genetic studies at sixteen to eighteen weeks of pregnancy. Amniotic fluid is extracted with a long hollow needle and fetal cells found in the fluid are cultured and examined. The culture takes about one month to grow, so there is a wait for test results. The test can tell parents the sex of the baby as well as identify over one hundred disorders, such as Tay-Sachs disease, Hunter's syndrome, neural-tube defects, Down's syndrome, and sickle-cell anemia. There are, however, a number of disorders that amniocentesis cannot detect.

Amniocentesis is not without some risk (possible infection, miscarriage, or damage to the baby and placenta) and is therefore not for everyone. Certain women are at greater risk of having a

baby with a defect and they would be likely candidates for amniocentesis. These women would include:

- those over thirty-five (statistically more likely to have a baby
  with Down's syndrome)
- those who already have one child with a genetic or chro-
  mosomal disease
- those who are carriers of Tay-Sachs or sickle-cell anemia
  and whose partners are as well
- those who, for medical reasons, need to be induced or delivered early by C-section (the test can gauge fetal lung
  maturity so the baby isn't taken out too soon)

CHORIONIC VILLI SAMPLING (CVS)

A thin catheter is inserted into the uterus through the vagina
and a small sampling of the chorionic villi, or fetal membrane,
is removed for study. CVS results are available faster than those
from amniocentesis, and the test can be done earlier in pregnancy, between the ninth and eleventh week. As with amniocentesis, there is a risk of miscarriage with CVS. It is important
to ask about the miscarriage rate for CVS and to use a good center
that has the best statistics. Because CVS is a relatively new procedure, amniocentesis is still more widely used. There are many
more centers that do amniocentesis. Finding skilled CVS tech-
nicians can be difficult in some areas. For this reason, it is tricky
to compare miscarriage rates for amniocentesis and CVS. In some
areas, the rate of miscarriage is higher with CVS than with amniocentesis, while in other areas it is the reverse.

The Patient-Practitioner Relationship

Once you've chosen a nurse-midwife or doctor, you need to form
a partnership of trust and mutual understanding. You can do this
by sharing information, asking questions, airing concerns.

If you read or hear advice that conflicts with something your caregiver has said, ask about it. Often there are justifiable reasons for different advice—you won't know until you ask.

If you are sick, in pain, or suspect a problem, say what's bothering you. Be as clear as you can. Unless you communicate, your provider can't know what you need. If the doctor or midwife doesn't listen to you, is always too rushed, or doesn't consider your concerns, get another health-care provider.

If you have a complaint, say so (for example, if you are repeatedly kept waiting for appointments due to overbooking). Conversely, a simple note of thanks for special help—spending extra time or returning 3:00 A.M. calls—is important, too. Let your nurse-midwife or doctor know you appreciate the time and interest.

When to Call Your Practitioner

During the pregnancy, you may occasionally experience some symptoms that should be brought to the attention of your physician or midwife. Your caregiver can then determine if your symptoms signal a medical problem or if they are no cause for alarm. For example, although bleeding during pregnancy can be a sign of miscarriage, many women bleed during pregnancy and then go on to deliver healthy, term babies.

As a general rule of thumb, your practitioner should be phoned any time you experience the following problems:

- vaginal bleeding or spotting (possible sign of miscarriage or ectopic pregnancy)
- abdominal pain (possible symptom of anything from impending miscarriage to urinary tract infection to fibroids on the uterus to a pulled muscle)
- severe vomiting (may or may not be pregnancy-related; see Chapter 5 for more on nausea and vomiting)
- fainting (any number of medical conditions may cause fainting, including—if accompanied by severe pain—ectopic pregnancy)

- blurred vision (may be one of the many symptoms of PIH, or pregnancy-induced hypertension)
- chronic headache pain (may be a sign of anything from tension to poor diet to high blood pressure. Most headaches respond to Tylenol, rest, and food; rarely, the headache is a sign of a serious medical condition, such as hypertension or PIH)
- sudden swelling (one of the symptoms of PIH)
- unusual vaginal discharge that itches, burns, or has an unpleasant odor (may be the sign of a vaginal infection)
- burning or bleeding upon urination (may be the sign of a urinary tract infection)
- dramatic decrease in or cessation of fetal movement (possible sign of fetal distress or fetal death)
- gush of water from the vagina (may be amniotic fluid and a sign of impending labor. If it occurs before the thirty-seventh week of pregnancy, it may be a sign of premature labor.)
- a concern that is nagging at you—why sit and wait and worry until the next appointment? (If you can, call during regular office hours.)

Not every pregnancy progresses smoothly and without incident from beginning to end. As the above list suggests, there are certain prenatal problems that may arise. The whole purpose of prenatal care is really to watch out for these complications and conditions. Most can be dealt with by your midwife. Some are better handled by a physician. If I feel that a problem has arisen that must be handled by a physician, I refer the woman to our backup doctor. Or, if she prefers, her prior obstetrician/ gynecologist is called if he or she has agreed to be a backup. If the problem is resolved prior to delivery, the obstetrician refers the patient back to me. This cooperative, team approach is very much appreciated by the families in my practice.

Unfortunately, there will be times when neither a midwife nor a physician will be able to offer you a solution. In the case of miscarriage, for example, nature often takes its course in spite of the best medical advice and knowledge. The point is that you should keep your practitioner informed but bear in mind that there may not always be an instant remedy for your pregnancy-related problem.

Miscarriage

Whether you call a midwife or a doctor about vaginal bleeding, both will begin by asking you the same questions:

How far along are you in this pregnancy?
Eighty-five percent of miscarriages occur in the first trimester. A late miscarriage, between twelve and twenty weeks or more, is more complicated because the fetus is better developed.

When did the bleeding start?
Bleeding that has been going on for six hours or more seems likely to end in miscarriage.

How heavy is the bleeding? How many pads per hour must you use?
Heavy bleeding means a miscarriage is more likely. Light spotting may resolve itself with bed rest.

What color is the blood—brown, red, or pink?
The blood of a miscarriage is usually bright red.

Is the bleeding accompanied by cramping or abdominal pain?
Bleeding in a miscarriage is likely to be accompanied by cramping.

Describe the pain (sharp, dull, rhythmic, constant, etc.). Where is the pain located?
If the pain is only on one side, it may be the sign of an ectopic pregnancy.

Was the bleeding accompanied by a gush of water?
In a late miscarriage, the fetus is surrounded by amniotic fluid. A gush of fluid would signal that the bag of waters has broken and a miscarriage is under way.

During the first trimester, unless there is heavy bleeding with strong cramping, a midwife will probably provide the care. Bleeding during pregnancy does not automatically mean unavoidable miscarriage. As many as 20 percent of women carrying to term have experienced some bleeding during their pregnancies. Since there is a chance that the bleeding will not end in miscarriage, a woman calling to complain of light to moderate bleeding will be put on bed rest by her midwife until the symptoms either go away or increase. Although bed rest may not seem medically sophisticated, it is really the best that can be offered women. It works in about one-third of the cases and is safer than the drugs that used to be given to prevent miscarriage. If the bleeding subsides, the woman is allowed to get up and slowly resume normal activities. She is also asked to come in for a checkup. At this visit, the practitioner can check for the baby's heartbeat, do a vaginal exam to see if the cervix has opened, and try to determine where the bleeding came from. In some cases, it's possible that the bleeding had nothing to do with the pregnancy but instead was the result of a polyp on the cervix or bad vaginitis that caused the vaginal wall to bleed.

If, on the other hand, the bleeding does not stop with bed rest, or if the bleeding and cramping are heavy, a miscarriage may be inevitable. In this case, it's often in the mother's best interest to move to the hospital rather than miscarry at home. This move, of course, will not prevent the miscarriage, but it may help the mother. Sometimes, fragments of the placenta remain and a D&C (dilatation and curettage) must be done to avoid the medical complications that can occur when a miscarriage is incomplete. This procedure is done by a physician in a hospital under local or general anesthesia. In a D&C the doctor dilates the cervix and scrapes the walls of the uterus clean, preventing further serious bleeding.

Early miscarriage is considered to be a type of natural selection process that is often better left unhampered. In other words, certain pregnancies spontaneously abort because the body seems to know naturally that the embryo was defective in some way. There is nothing anyone can do to stop this from happening. Hormones are no longer used to prolong the pregnancy because they can cause fetal abnormalities. I have seen a number of patients through early miscarriages and I know how threatening it is to feel that your baby is dying and that no one can help you. Although it is a lonely time, you are not alone in your experience. Early miscarriages are extremely common. Many women have them without ever realizing it—they know only that they had a late and heavy period. A miscarriage does not mean that you are not healthy or that you won't be able to go on to carry a healthy baby to term.

Whenever a woman is miscarrying, I always tell her plainly, "Your baby has died. I'm very sorry." Often this is the only time she hears the phrase "Your baby has died." Usually, she hears terms such as "blighted ovum," "embryo," "products of conception," or "miscarriage." Most people, including many doctors and nurses, feel uncomfortable with the grief process and avoid talking with the mother about her feelings. Most people either say nothing to the woman about the miscarriage or make a well-meaning remark like "You'll get pregnant again." A woman needs time to grieve over the loss of *this* baby before she can think about another pregnancy.

Women who miscarry need to know that they did not do anything to cause the miscarriage. Women have told me all kinds of things that they think they did to cause the miscarriage, from having intercourse to exercising to catching a cold. I have even heard from women that they didn't want the baby at first and that the baby knew this and died. None of these things can cause a miscarriage.

Women who are further along at the time of miscarriage will have an even harder time recovering emotionally because the bonding process has progressed and the expectations are bigger. I explain to them that the emotional recovery process does not always follow a steady path. Women may think they've gotten over the miscarriage until they see a still-pregnant woman with an obviously similar due date or until their old due date comes along. Knowing that this may happen helps a woman cope.

Anyone who miscarries repeatedly (two or three times in a row) needs to be assessed to determine the problem. Obstetricians/gynecologists specializing in fertility problems or high-risk pregnancies are best qualified to help these women carry babies to term.

Ectopic Pregnancy

Symptoms include severe abdominal pain (usually one-sided), fainting, and vaginal bleeding.

Of all women who experience bleeding during the first trimester, a few may be experiencing ectopic pregnancies. An ectopic pregnancy is a tubal pregnancy. The egg normally implants itself in the wall of the uterus, but in an ectopic pregnancy the egg implants itself in the fallopian tube. If it grows in the tube for much longer than ten weeks, the tube explodes, causing life-threatening hemorrhaging. The condition is very rare but more common in women who've had surgery on their tubes, or tubal infections, or who've used an IUD for a long time.

If a woman has this history and if the pain she is experiencing is mainly on one side, she needs a sonogram and a series of blood tests for HCG (human chorionic gonadotropin). A woman who has frequent episodes of spotting may also need a sonogram, as spotting too can be a sign of an ectopic pregnancy. The sonogram will usually give a picture of where the embryo is implanted, and the blood tests for HCG will help confirm the suspicion of ectopic pregnancy. An ectopic pregnancy must be removed surgically by a physician, through an abdominal incision. Unfortunately, this surgery always results in the loss of the fallopian tube on that side, but women can still get pregnant, since the tube on the other side is intact.

Ectopic pregnancies are both physically and emotionally traumatic for the woman and her family. At the Maternity Center we provide close support for our clients throughout this difficult time. The follow-up visits are done by both the physicians and the nurse-midwives, each of us contributing our expertise for the benefit of the patient.

Urinary Tract Infection (UTI)

Urinary tract infections occur more frequently in pregnant women than in nonpregnant women. Cystitis, a bladder infection, is the most common type of urinary tract infection. Symptoms include blood in the urine, pain on urination, pain over the bladder area, increased frequency of urination, back pain (which may suggest a more serious infection with kidney involvement), extreme fatigue, chills, and fever.

All urinary tract infections deserve prompt attention and treatment with antibiotics. Since untreated infections can cause premature labor and kidney damage, it is very important that any possibility of UTI be looked into with a urinalysis and culture. Most respond well to oral antibiotics and can be treated by your nurse-midwife. A physician is consulted when there are complicating circumstances.

Vaginal Infections

Vaginal infections are also common during pregnancy. They can be treated by your physician or nurse-midwife with vaginal or oral medications that will not harm your baby. Below is information on the various types of infections.

Monilia: (also called candida, or yeast infection). Symptoms include itching and a discharge resembling cottage cheese. The odor is not foul but strong. It is most common in the summer months. Monilia should be treated. If the baby is born while you have this infection, it can cause thrush (a monilia infection in the mouth of the baby). Thrush is not considered dangerous, but it is a nuisance and the baby must then be treated with antifungal oral medications. The woman is treated with a vaginal cream or suppository such as Monistat, Gyne-Lotrimin, or Nystatin.

Trichomoniasis: This is a sexually transmitted infection; symptoms include odor, itchiness, and a bubbly, watery discharge. The infection is usually treated with a specific drug called Flagyl in nonpregnant women, but there is some question as to whether or not the drug should be used during pregnancy. Unfortunately, it is really the only thing that will stop the infection. Betadyne gel, however, can be prescribed to at least help get rid of some of the symptoms until after the birth when you can safely take Flagyl. On the positive side, trichomoniasis has no known effect on babies.

Group B streptococci: Symptoms are few and difficult to spot, so many health-care providers routinely take a culture in the eighth month of pregnancy. This organism has been implicated in the premature rupture of membranes and infection of newborns with sepsis (a potentially life-threatening infection). If diagnosed in the mother, group B streptococci can be treated with oral antibiotics, thereby preventing infection in the newborn.

Chlamydia: This sexually transmitted organism, harbored within the cervix, produces few reliable signs and symptoms in the mother. Chlamydia can cause an eye infection in the newborn (chlamydia conjunctivitis) and pneumonia and so is often routinely tested for and treated prior to delivery.

Gardnerella: This bacterial infection in the vagina produces increased discharge, odor, possible itching and burning. Clinically it's similar to a head cold—if you treat it, it may go away; if you don't treat it, it may go away. Usually, your body can fight it off alone. If symptoms persist or worsen, however, the infection can be treated with antibiotics.

Fibroids of the Uterus

Fibroids are muscle tumors that can grow inside or on the outside of the uterus (a muscular organ). They are almost always benign (not cancerous) and often grow during pregnancy. They can range in size from a few inches in diameter to the size of a grapefruit or larger. Fibroids can cause abdominal pain and burning sensations. They are easily diagnosed by sonogram. Most fibroids cause only minor problems during pregnancy and shrink considerably after birth. Occasionally, however, they can become so large that they can obstruct labor. In some cases, surgery is required, usually performed after delivery.

Pregnancy-Induced Hypertension (PIH)

Symptoms of PIH include swelling, a sudden jump in weight gain, protein in the urine, headache, high blood pressure, and hyperreflexia (reflexes like the knee jerk are more pronounced than usual). PIH, also known as eclampsia or toxemia, can be life-threatening if untreated. When treated early and aggressively, it can be controlled. Severe eclampsia can result in seizures, growth retardation in the fetus, and hypoxia (decreased flow of oxygen to the fetus). Women at highest risk for PIH are first-time mothers in their early teens and first-time mothers over age thirty-five. The overall incidence of PIH in the population is 5 percent. Early detection is the key, so at each visit during your pregnancy your urine will be tested for protein, your blood pressure and weight gain will be recorded, and your practitioner will look for swelling. Swelling and weight gain are part of normal pregnancy and become worrisome only if they are excessive or combined with other symptoms. There is still some disagreement as to how toxemia can be prevented or treated, because the cause of toxemia is still a mystery. Doctors used to advise restricted weight gain, restricted salt intake, restricted fluid intake, and the use of diuretics. None of these things worked. Changing to a high-protein, low-carbohydrate diet and encouraging the woman to lie on her left side and drink eight large glasses of water a day seem to work when the symptoms are mild to moderate. Hospitalization becomes necessary if these measures don't work. Drugs to control the high blood pressure are also prescribed in moderate to severe PIH.

A woman with moderate or severe PIH cannot deliver at home or in a birth center. Hospitals have the technology and drugs that are essential for the safe management of these mothers and their babies. A physician usually manages the pregnancy and birth in these cases, while the nurse-midwife continues to offer counseling and support.

Premature Labor and Birth

Premature labor is defined as labor that begins before the thirty-seventh week of pregnancy. Be alert to the signs of premature labor and call your practitioner anytime you experience menstruallike cramps, low back pain that comes and goes in waves, cramping in the thighs, any vaginal spotting or bleeding or increased mucous discharge, water leaking from the vagina (rupture of membranes), or contractions that are regular. Your midwife or doctor will examine you to determine whether or not you are in labor and whether there have been any changes in the cervix. You may then be placed on bed rest to see if the symptoms will subside on their own. Depending upon the situation, you may instead be hospitalized or given medications to relax the uterus and prevent premature birth. In some cases, stitches are placed in the cervix to keep it closed. For very early delivery, the care of an obstetrician is essential for the best outcome for mother and baby. If your local hospital doesn't have an intensive-care nursery, you will probably be moved so that you can deliver in one that does have these facilities. For a very premature delivery, the obstetrician may elect to deliver the baby by cesarean in an effort to reduce any birth trauma a vaginal delivery might place on a very immature baby.

High-risk nursery care has dramatically changed the outcomes for premature babies. Your newborn can be cared for with the most up-to-date medical knowledge available. The outlook for babies born too soon is constantly improving.

Abruptio Placenta

A very rare and very serious bleeding problem known as abruptio placenta can occur during pregnancy. In this disorder, the placenta begins to separate from the wall of the uterus, causing a life-threatening hemorrhage for both mother and fetus. Delivery is often by cesarean section. Although maternal death from bleeding is quite rare, the rate of death of the baby is quite high (35 percent). Women with high blood pressure are at greater risk for abruptio placenta. Because of the serious emergency nature of abruptio placenta, it is always managed by a physician.

Placenta Previa

The placenta normally implants itself at the top, or fundus, of the uterus. When it implants low in the uterus, near or over the cervix, it can cause bleeding during the last half of the pregnancy and/or during labor. Depending on how much of the cervix is covered by the placenta, bleeding will range from mild to severe. Early diagnosis of placenta previa by sonogram is common, and in most of those cases, the situation will resolve itself by the end of the pregnancy. This self-correction occurs because of the growth of the uterus below the site where the placenta is implanted, so that the placenta no longer covers the cervix.

If the placenta covers the whole cervix (complete placenta previa) at the time of delivery, cesarean section is the only safe method of delivery. Partial placenta previa or low lying placentas may cause only minimal bleeding and vaginal delivery can be tried under careful monitoring in the hospital. Because of the serious nature of placenta previa, it is always managed either jointly by nurse-midwife and physician or totally by the physician.

Twins

The news of a twin pregnancy (or triplet, quadruplet, etc.) is often met with a mixture of shock, delight, dismay, and even fear. With the availability of sonograms, most multiple births are now diagnosed well in advance of labor.

During pregnancy, a woman carrying multiple fetuses will usually experience an increase in the "normal discomforts" of pregnancy, due to the extra size and weight of two babies, two placentas, and more amniotic fluid. There may be more swelling, heartburn, backache, and varicose veins, for example. The expectant mother is also more prone to anemia and fatigue. Because of the overstretched uterus, a woman with a multiple pregnancy is more apt to go into premature labor. She may therefore have to be put on bed rest and/or medications if she starts to show signs of premature labor.

Twin delivery is considered high-risk. The concern is for the well-being of the second twin. After delivery of the first baby, the placenta may start to detach in response to the change in uterine size and the second baby's oxygen supply can be compromised. The hospital delivery room should be used because of the increased risk of complications.

On the positive side, twin children are special people, be they identical or fraternal. During their first few months of life, the new mother should try to get as much extra help as possible, for raising two babies simultaneously involves a monumental amount of work. There are a number of support groups to help parents plan for and deal with the unique aspects of raising multiples. The experiences of other parents can be a source of wisdom, comfort, and commonsense advice, especially for first-time parents.

4

Eating for Two

Midwives have always emphasized good nutrition as the key to a healthy pregnancy and baby. Unfortunately, nutritional issues are often rushed through by doctors or overlooked by patients. Nutrition is an important aspect of good prenatal care. Your eating habits have a direct effect on your baby's size and health. Don't despair if you have a sweet tooth, however. Even if you love junk food, you are not destined for nutritional failure. You can still learn to satisfy all your nutritional needs. This chapter will give the answers to your specific nutrition questions, including tips and tricks you'll *want* to know about! Even if you are nutritionally illiterate, you are not a hopeless case. You *can* learn to make the nutritional changes that pregnancy demands.

First, take an honest look at your normal eating patterns. You may have no idea how good or bad your diet actually is until you do so. Keep a food diary to determine what you eat during an average day. Food can be separated into four basic groups: dairy products; meat and protein; fruits and vegetables; and breads and cereals. Look at your diary after a few days. Does your diet include red meats? Cheeses of any kind? Chicken? Fish? Eggs? Rice, beans, or potatoes? Fresh fruit? Whole grain cereal or breads? Green vegetables? Yellow vegetables? Do you take any dietary supplements (wheat germ, soy, vitamins, etc.)? Do you drink milk? Water? Coffee or tea? Soda? Are you on a special diet of any kind? (If so, be sure to tell your CNM or doctor.) Do you eat potato chips, candy bars? Check your list against the information in this chapter. Share your findings with your midwife to learn more about how to improve your pregnancy diet and to find out just how these improvements can be made. If you know very little about good nutritional habits, you'll want to spend some time discussing your current diet with your midwife or doctor.

Nutritional Guidelines

Nutritional guidelines can be more difficult in the abstract than in reality, so before we get into the technicalities of the recommended daily allowances for pregnant women, let's look at a sample menu so you can see how easy it is to achieve good nutrition.

Sample Menu

This sample day's menu should give you a good idea of how you can fill your daily nutritional requirements.

BREAKFAST

Orange juice or ½ grapefruit
1 or 2 eggs
Whole-wheat toast
Milk

LUNCH

Meat or cheese sandwich on
    whole-wheat bread
Salad with cabbage, tomato,
    spinach, lettuce, carrots
Glass of milk or ½ cup yogurt

SNACK

Apple
Whole-wheat crackers
Cheese

DINNER

Broiled chicken or fish
Squash
Salad
Potatoes or rice
Glass of milk

Pregnancy calls for additional energy and nutritional requirements. You need to make dietary changes in order to compensate
for the increased maternal work associated with the growth of
the fetus and placenta. According to the Food and Nutrition
Board, National Academy of Sciences (the group that determines
the recommended daily allowances for men and women), pregnant women daily need *more* of the following:

> 30 more grams of *protein* for a total of 76 grams
>
> 1,000 more IU of *vitamin A* for a total of 5,000 IU
>
> 20 more mg of *vitamin C* for a total of 80 mg
>
> 200 more IU of *vitamin D* for a total of 400–600 IU
>
> 0.6 more mg of *vitamin B_6* for a total of 2.6 mg
>
> 0.4 more mg of *thiamine* for a total of 1.5 mg
>
> 0.3 more mg of *riboflavin* for a total of 1.5 mg
>
> 400 more mg of *calcium* for a total of 1,200 mg
>
> 400 more mg of *phosphorus* for a total of 1,200 mg
>
> 30–60 mg of *iron* supplement
>
> 5 more mg of *zinc* for a total of 20 mg
>
> 150 more mg of *magnesium* for a total of 450 mg
>
> 25 more mcg of *iodine* for a total of 175 mcg
>
> 300–350 more *calories* for a total of 2,400 calories

Now I Know That I Should Eat More Protein, Calcium, Vitamins, and Minerals Every Day. But Where Do These Things Come From?

Pregnant women often know what they are supposed to eat,
but most have little idea of which foods fall into which categories.
Here's a simple list.

Protein: milk, yogurt, cheese, meat, fish, eggs, beans, lentils,
peas, nuts, tofu

Carbohydrates: bread, cereal, pasta, rice, potatoes, bananas

Fats: butter and oil

Folic acid: brewer's yeast, kidney, liver, brains, bran, peas, endive, broccoli, spinach, nuts, whole grains

Vitamin A: carrots, parsley, leafy green vegetables, liver, dairy products

Vitamin B: yeast, whole-grain cereals, liver, eggs, bran, dairy products, fish, nuts, dried fruit

Vitamin C: oranges and other citrus fruits, red peppers, green peppers, tomatoes, watercress

Vitamin D: milk, dairy products, spinach, parsley, dried figs, almonds, watercress, liver, herrings, sardines

Vitamin E: vegetable oils, cereals, meat, eggs, milk, wheat germ, nuts

Vitamin B_6: grains, wheat germ, bran, nuts, seeds, legumes, corn

Niacin: pork, peanuts, beans, peas

Thiamine: pork, beef, liver, whole grains, legumes

Calcium: cheese, milk, yogurt, spinach, parsley, dried figs, nuts, watercress, soy flour, egg yolk

Iron: liver, lean meat, bran, wheat germ, parsley, dried fruit, egg yolk, prunes, beans, lentils

Zinc: meat, liver, eggs, oysters

Magnesium: nuts, green vegetables, whole grains, dried beans and peas

Now you know where to find the right nutrients and how much of each you need. But do you know how your body uses these nutrients and calories?

What Good Nutrition Does for You and Your Baby

Here is a breakdown of some of the ways your body uses all this good food.

Calories: Three hundred calories is the extra amount you need to compensate for the energy drain of increased maternal blood volume and fetal and placental growth. Calories provide energy for tissue building. The increase in the number of calories is not great, so make sure that you are selecting high-protein, high-calcium, iron-rich foods that are low in calories. If you do, you will stay within the suggested 2,400-calorie range and still get all the nutrients you need. Don't pad your diet with sugary treats to meet the additional calorie requirement. Remember also that these figures are based on averages. Your specific prepregnant weight, your baby's weight, your appetite, your metabolism, and other factors may all affect your particular caloric intake. These figures are meant only as general guidelines. Everyone gains weight differently from the same amount of food, making it difficult to give everyone the same caloric requirements and expect the same outcome.

Protein: The meat, fish, and poultry you eat during your pregnancy help to build and repair tissues. They also supply energy and help your body in the development of the placenta, amniotic fluid, and extra blood. Protein requirements are greater in the last trimester as your baby grows larger.

Calcium and Phosphorus: Calcium and phosphorus help build bones and teeth. As with protein, calcium requirements are greater in the last trimester because of the baby's increased size.

Vitamin D: This vitamin is necessary for absorption of the calcium and phosphorus.

Iron: Iron combined with protein makes hemoglobin. The mother's iron supply is used by the fetus to form his or her own iron supply. An iron supplement is usually recommended during pregnancy, especially in the last six weeks when fetal requirements are greater.

Zinc: The zinc in the meat, eggs, and seafood you eat helps your baby's skeleton and nervous system to form properly.

Magnesium: Magnesium promotes tissue growth and neuromuscular development.

Vitamin A: The green and yellow vegetables you eat contain vitamin A, which helps the growth of bones, tissues, and cells. It also provides for healthy skin and mucous membranes.

Vitamin E: This vitamin is needed for tissue growth and healthy red blood cells.

Vitamin C: The citrus fruits you eat contain vitamin C, which helps form tissues and aids in the body's absorption of iron.

How Do I Ensure a Good Diet?

Balance is the key. The more we learn about nutrition, the more evident it is that all of the vitamins, minerals, proteins, and fats that make up our diet must come from a variety of sources.

For those who know little about nutrition and glaze over when reading chapters like this one, I have *one* piece of advice *only*: *shop the periphery of your grocery store.* This is where you will usually find the fresh foods that are best for you: the fresh fruits and vegetables, dairy products, breads, meat, chicken, and fish. In the center aisles, you tend to find the processed items that are not so terrific: cookies, canned goods, potato chips, cake mixes, etc. So this one simple tip may be all you need to guarantee a great diet without having to understand fully the ins and outs of nitrites and nutrients. Here are just a few more simple pieces of nutritional wisdom to keep in mind:

Try one new vegetable and fruit every week. This will counteract your natural inclination to eat the same trusted food over and over with no variation.

Shop by color. As you wheel through the fresh-produce section, select one red, one orange, one green, one yellow, one white vegetable. Throw them all together in a salad or chop up some and toss them in with your meals.

Buy the freshest foods available. The fresher the food, the higher the nutrient level. Canned and frozen foods have little good stuff (vitamins, nutrients) left in them.

Wash your produce! All fruits and vegetables must be washed thoroughly to rinse off the chemicals that are sprayed on crops. Even "organically grown" produce should be washed. It may not have been sprayed with chemicals but was still grown in ground that contains chemicals. These days, it's almost impossible to find any completely "untainted" foods.

Add pasta to a salad. Try spinach or whole-wheat pastas for added nutritional value.

Eat red meats, poultry, and fish. They are excellent sources of the protein you need. But remember: although red meat is high in protein, it's also high in fat, so don't eat too much of it. Chicken and fish are much leaner sources of protein.

Include other wonderful sources of protein such as beans, legumes, cheese, tofu, pasta, nuts, pork, ham, lamb, shellfish, and eggs. Vegetarians often rely on beans and legumes for their protein. To make these a "complete protein," however, you'll have to add yogurt or eggs. If you are on a vegetarian diet, check with a nutritionist familiar with vegetarian diets for advice.

Steam your vegetables. If vegetables are boiled in water, all the vitamins go into the water (and the water usually gets thrown out!).

Choose whole-grain breads and cereals, not white bread or sugar-coated cereals. This means breads that are made with whole wheat and wheat germ. Also try rye and pumpernickel breads.

For those who aren't used to whole-grain breads, try oatmeal bread—you'll like the taste, and it's better for you than white breads.

Buy a vegetarian cookbook even if you're a meat-eater. It may help you to find creative, tasty recipes for vegetables. Simple steamed veggies can be hard to force down if you're normally a nonvegetable eater.

Avoid additives. Processed lunch meats, for example, contain additives to keep them from spoiling. Your own baked or boiled chicken makes better sandwich meat than packaged processed chicken slices.

Add bean sprouts, cucumber, carrot shavings, tomatoes, and cheese to your sandwiches for added nutritional punch.

How Can I Make This Seasick Feeling Go Away?

For most women, nausea lasts "only" through the sixteenth week. Then it disappears as mysteriously as it arrived. Those sixteen weeks can seem like a lifetime, though! Commonly called "morning sickness," nausea and vomiting can really occur at any time of the day (all day for some women). Other women sail through their pregnancies without feeling the slightest bit sick. No one knows why different women react differently or why feelings of nausea can vary in intensity from pregnancy to pregnancy in the same woman. On the bright side, nausea is not a bad sign. In fact, it is a good one—an indication that pregnancy hormones are high and that this is a stable, healthy pregnancy. If you're really feeling sick, this news will cheer you up only for a short time (maybe five minutes), so I'm including a list of twenty-two things you can try to counteract that nauseated feeling. None of these is certain to work, but there's a chance you'll find something here that will do the trick for you:

1. Stop taking your prenatal vitamins for a while. Sometimes they make nausea worse. It is better to skip the vitamins

and be able to eat well than to take the vitamins and vomit.

2. Keep something in your stomach at all times. Don't go more than an hour without having a small snack. Hunger makes the nausea worse.

3. Stash crackers, dry cereal, and dry toast, both at work and in your purse. They'll usually stay down and are convenient to have with you at all times.

4. Prepare foods that *do not have a strong odor*. Foods that must bake for a long time in the oven and that fill the house with the odor of cooked food will probably bother you a lot more than a simple sandwich or cold salad.

5. For now, find whatever you *can* eat and go for it, even if it is not the best thing nutritionally.

6. For now, stop eating foods that make you feel sick, even if it is a food, like milk, that you know is "good for you."

7. Avoid greasy foods and fried foods.

8. Try a vitamin B_6 supplement (about 20 mg a day), but check with your doctor or midwife first.

9. Have a snack right before you go to sleep so you don't wake up empty in the morning.

10. Have some food by your bed so you can eat something before you get up in the morning. Get up very slowly, sitting first to eat something. If you bound out of bed on an empty stomach, you're more likely to feel sick.

11. Get someone else to do the shopping and prepare the meals. (For most of us, this is the impossible dream, but it may be worth a try.)

12. Rest. If you're tired, you're more likely to be nauseated.

13. Drink a glass of milk before bed.

14. Try ginger tea. Boil ginger root in water, strain, and drink with some added honey for flavor. Some women swear by this remedy.

15. Try peppermint tea.

16. Try raspberry-leaf tea.

17. Try a high-protein diet: tuna fish, eggs, low-fat milk, peanut butter.

18. If that doesn't work, try a high-carbohydrate diet: pastas, rice, baked potaoes, bananas, dry toast, muesli.
19. Drink warm milk mixed with wheat germ. Sip a few teaspoons each hour.
20. Avoid fatty foods.
21. Try a diet of just one food that you seem to tolerate well. Add one other food the next day, and so on, until you find a balanced diet of a few things that don't make you sick.
22. On the subject of spicy foods: contrary to logic, some women find that extremely spicy foods (Indian, Szechwan) go down more easily than other foods. This, of course, conflicts with the notion that foods with a strong odor should be avoided, but if it works for you, who cares?

I've Tried Everything But I Can't Keep Much Food Down. How Will the Baby Survive?

If nausea is preventing you from eating a balanced diet, don't worry. The baby's needs right now are small. During the first few months, the baby can draw on the mother's nutritional stores if necessary.

Am I Gaining Too Much/Too Little Weight?

The quality of your diet is much more important than the number of pounds you gain. Weight gain depends on your size and stature, as well as on the size of your baby and the placenta that supports it.

Generally, total weight gain in pregnancy is between twenty-five and thirty pounds, but it may vary from a low of twenty to a high of forty pounds or more. Here's how the weight is distributed:

7–8 lbs.: baby

1–2 lbs.: placenta

2 lbs.:   uterus

2 lbs.:   amniotic fluid

2 lbs.:   breasts

3 lbs.:   increased blood volume

4 lbs.:   fluid

7½ lbs.:   extra body fat and protein stores

28–30 lbs.:   total

During the first trimester, most women gain about five pounds. This is an average. Don't be alarmed if you gain nothing during the first three months or, conversely, if you gain a lot more than five pounds. A large weight gain in the early months is sometimes due to twins or excessive water retention, but more commonly the pregnancy is single and normal. The mother is just eating more calories than she is burning off. It's that simple! Many women have sedentary jobs and many rarely exercise. When pregnant, they rightly add recommended starch, protein, and dairy products and may begin to gain weight at what they find to be an alarming rate! The answer is to cut out some of the high-calorie foods, such as junk foods and desserts, and to get more of your protein from chicken and fish than from red meats. Also, by increasing your exercise (within reason, of course), you'll be able to burn off some of the extra calories.

If you were overweight before the pregnancy, you still need to gain weight during pregnancy. Now is not the time to diet or fast. However, you needn't gain forty pounds; keep the weight gain to twenty-five pounds, if possible. The most important criterion is a well-balanced diet. A number of my overweight patients go to the Weight Watchers program for pregnant women. This excellent program is designed to keep pregnancy weight gain down while maintaining a nutritionally healthy diet for mother and baby.

Weight gain usually increases in the second and third trimesters. Most women gain about one pound a week after the first three months. Some women find themselves gaining much more. Women who gain a total of sixty pounds do not have healthier babies than women who gain twenty-five pounds, and obesity *can be* a major health concern. Moderate weight gain of twenty-five to thirty-five pounds has been shown to produce the best outcomes for mother and baby.

Occasionally, a woman comes to me who has trouble gaining weight. Although it's hard for dieters like myself to believe, some women just don't have much of an appetite and eat very little or like to eat very low-calorie foods. I cared for one woman who was having lots of problems gaining weight. She claimed that she ate to the point of being stuffed at each meal. When I delved into her food habits and had her keep a diary recording what her meals consisted of, I found that she was eating almost nothing but spinach salads. This woman was eating pounds of spinach each week, which was a great iron supply but provided almost no calories! I recommended an Italian restaurant in the area and told her to have a pasta entrée several times a week. She gained!

Nongainers need to increase their calories and decrease exercise, and they will gain weight. I promise. High-calorie nutritious foods include cheese, whole milk, ice cream (made with real milk and cream), beef, pasta, bread, peanut butter and jelly. Make a big twelve-ounce milkshake every day for a snack with ice cream, milk, eggs, and real fruit (strawberries or bananas, for instance) and you'll gain. Add whole milk to casseroles and soups. Decrease exercise by walking instead of running, or swimming fewer laps at a slower pace.

Should I Take Prenatal Vitamins and Iron?

Most people who care for pregnant women advise taking prenatal vitamins with iron and folic acid during the pregnancy. Lack of folic acid has been associated with spinal cord defects (such as spina bifida, which is characterized by failure of the spinal cord to close normally). Iron has been shown to prevent anemia in women during pregnancy. Both iron and folic acid are found in the foods we eat.

Vitamin pills haven't been shown to do much; it has been difficult to demonstrate any difference in the outcomes of women who took vitamins and those who did not. Prenatal vitamins in the prescribed doses have never been shown to harm anyone, however, and so are often offered as a supplement to a good diet. They should never be a replacement for a good diet. Sometimes, women who experience nausea have difficulty taking prenatal vitamins that contain a lot of iron. The iron can be too hard for them to digest. It can also cause constipation, so be sure to eat plenty of bran if this seems to be a problem for you. Talk with your caregiver about lower iron doses.

I Hate Milk. How Can I Get Enough Calcium?

Women who don't drink milk because they don't like the taste should add some of the following foods to their diet:

cheese

yogurt

broccoli

canned sardines

salmon

collard greens

mustard or turnip greens

sesame seeds

ice cream (if made with real milk and cream) or ice milk

powdered skim milk (can be added to casseroles and the milk you drink to give one cup of milk the calcium equivalent of two) skim milk added to soups, sauces, casseroles (the taste of the milk is hidden by the food)

Women who eat few dairy products of any kind or who are allergic to milk need to take supplemental calcium beyond what is in prenatal vitamins.

Many pediatricians and allergists believe that if a woman has already had a child with an allergy to cow's milk, she should limit her intake of dairy products during the next pregnancy and lactation. The theory is that there is less chance of the baby developing an allergy to milk when exposed to it later in life. You may want to ask about this.

I'm a Candy, Cake, and Cookie Freak. Am I Hurting My Baby?

Candy, cake, and cookies generally contain empty calories, so before you indulge make sure you are eating very well and not gaining too much weight. Will these foods hurt your baby? No. Will they help? No.

To satisfy that urge for sweet baked goods, try something that has some nutritional value as well, such as cornbread, oatmeal-raisin cookies, or an apple crisp with raisins and sunflower seeds. Carrot cake, banana bread (easy on the sugar), milkshakes, fruit in yogurt, and pumpkin pie, for example, can all satisfy a sweet tooth without being quite as nutritionally empty as a store-bought candy bar.

Should I Avoid Salt?

Salt is necessary for health, but it must be used in moderation. Use a little in your cooking if you like, but don't pour on any extra at the table. Eliminate foods that are high in salt, such as ham, potato chips, pickles, and bacon. Heavy doses can cause excessive water retention and high blood pressure, whether you're pregnant or not. For more on water retention, see the section on edema in Chapter 5.

What's Wrong with Drinking Alcohol During Pregnancy?

Consuming large amounts of alcohol (six to eight alcoholic drinks a day) can cause problems with mental and physical growth in the fetus. This is called fetal alcohol syndrome. Some of the problems that have been associated with this condition include mental retardation, altered facial characteristics, and small body size. Remember, alcohol is a drug.

What about moderate drinking or occasional drinking? Moderate drinking (one or two drinks per day) doesn't usually produce fetal alcohol syndrome, but it does constantly expose the baby to a drug that can cause serious problems. Each baby will react slightly differently to the alcohol in your system. Why take chances? Be good to yourself and mother your baby from the start—change that drinking pattern. An occasional glass of liquor (wine or beer once or twice a month) has not been shown to harm a developing baby. So if it's a celebration you joined in with a toast, don't get hysterical thinking you may have harmed your baby with one drink. That's going to extremes. Just use good judgment.

What if you had several drinks before you knew you were pregnant? This happens a lot. Women ask me about this all the time. Fortunately, before you miss a period the fertilized egg has not yet developed a placenta and is therefore not yet connected to the mother's circulatory system in any way. So any drugs, caffeine, or alcohol you took can't cross to the developing embryo and cause problems. Just about the time a woman realizes she is pregnant, the placenta develops. So you needn't worry about the drinks you had in the first weeks after conception.

How Bad Is Caffeine?

Large amounts of caffeine have been associated with birth defects in animal studies. It is less clear whether there is a cause-and-effect relationship in humans between caffeine and birth defects or between caffeine and other problems such as prematurity or stillbirths. But caffeine is a drug and it is often ingested daily by women in the form of coffee, tea, and colas. My advice? The less caffeine you drink, the better. You may be interested to know that coffee has more caffeine in it than tea and that tea contains more than colas do. If you have trouble giving up your favorite caffeinated drink completely, don't panic. One cup of coffee is better than five. Since caffeine has been proved harmful only in very large quantities, don't lose sleep over this one. You needn't start building up guilt before the baby is even born. Guilt and motherhood do not have to be synonymous.

My Mother Smoked When She Was Pregnant with Me and I'm Fine. Why Can't I Smoke Now That I'm Pregnant?

Although it is tempting to look back at the "good old days" and all the things our mothers were allowed to do during their pregnancies (drink alcohol, take aspirin, smoke cigarettes), it is much smarter to look at what research is telling us now. And what research tells us is that *smoking decreases the oxygen supply to the baby* and statistically is related to lower-birth-weight babies.

Being a former smoker myself, I do understand how you feel about the joys of smoking and I know how hard it is to break the habit. If it weren't so bad for my health and that of those around me, I would probably be smoking right now as I write this book. But I know that smoking can cause cancer, emphysema, bronchitis, bad breath, and yellow teeth, so I don't do it. Pregnant women have even more reason to quit or cut down.

Besides the health problems they cause themselves, their babies are getting less oxygen.

Some women claim they smoke to keep their weight under control. I think this is a lousy excuse. There are many other ways to keep your weight under control that are a lot better for you and your baby.

Face it: kicking the habit is hard to do. Most people need help. There are often programs you can join at your local hospital, or you can contact a group called Smokenders. Don't rule out less traditional methods that may help you: hypnosis works wonders for some people. If you can't quit, cut back. Cutting back is a lot better than continuing to smoke a pack a day. It's tough but not impossible. You can do it.

What If I Get a Cold or a Headache? Can't I Take Anything for It?

The general rule of thumb I give is to avoid all medications while you're pregnant unless you really need them. If you're not sure about the safety of a particular medication, ask your health-care provider or pharmacist about it. Remember, even if it's sold over the counter, it may still be dangerous for you. Always check with your doctor or midwife first. Aspirin, for example, is the most commonly used nonprescription drug and should be avoided during pregnancy. (Tylenol usually works as well as aspirin and is considered safer.) If you purchase a cold medicine, read the label—it often contains aspirin and alcohol as well.

If you have an ongoing medical problem such as migraines, eczema, or asthma, ask what medicines are safe to use, preferably even before you get pregnant. If you develop a medical problem and end up in the emergency room or a doctor's office, remind everyone there that you are pregnant. If a medication or treatment is presribed, ask if it is safe to take during pregnancy. Don't assume they remember you're pregnant even if you wrote it on your medical form. You must check out the safety of any medication or procedures prescribed.

What About Recreational Drugs?

Cocaine, marijuana, and other so-called recreational drugs are not safe during pregnancy or at any other time. In the case of cocaine, the baby gets the first "hit" soon after the mother does. To make matters worse, the baby excretes the drug through his or her kidneys into the amniotic fluid. Fetuses drink amniotic fluid and so get repeated doses of cocaine until it is finally excreted via the mother's bloodstream. Cocaine is lethal—it can cause strokes and heart attacks in unborn and newborn babies. Those who survive go through withdrawal. If you're on a drug, you can get help. Be honest and tell your doctor or midwife about your habit. They'll connect you with the right resources so you can find a way to change your life and protect your baby.

How Much Water Should I Drink?

During pregnancy you want to be sure to get enough fluids. Water is essential for your good health and good nutrition: it carries nutrients to your cells and carries waste products away. It also aids digestion and helps regulate your body temperature. Aim for at least two quarts a day (eight to ten glasses). Instead of nonstop water, you can also drink unsweetened fruit and vegetable juices. One reason you need so many glasses of water while you're pregnant is because it provides fluid for your increased blood volume and for the amniotic fluid your body makes. (Besides water, you should also drink another two or three glasses of milk or make sure your diet includes its calcium equivalent.)

Are Herbal Remedies a Real Alternative or Black Magic?

Doctors, midwives, and mothers sometimes use herbal remedies and treatments for pregnancy and childbirth. Some people find that these herbs work quite well. Others are suspicious of them. Without a doubt, however, herbs are potent. About half of all our prescription drugs come from herbs. Aspirin, for example, comes from willows.

Although herbs sound like they may provide the ideal answer to life's discomforts and ailments, they should be treated with the same respect we give drugs. In other words, some can be dangerous if used incorrectly or in the wrong doses. Herbs are not necessarily any safer just because they're "natural." You should always check with your pregnancy caregiver, a homeopathic physician, or an herbalist before self-treating with herbs.

Here are some of the common herbs women sometimes use in pregnancy.

Chamomile

Spearmint

Ginger

Wormwood

Raspberry leaf

Used as teas, all of these are said to help battle nausea in pregnant women. Raspberry-leaf tea has also been associated with easier labors. It supposedly prepares the cervix for delivery and is said to increase the effectiveness of uterine contractions in labor.

Lemon verbena

Chamomile

Cinnamon

Cloves

Ginger

Nutmeg

Peppermint

Caraway

All of these are said to help curb heartburn and indigestion.

Blue cohosh

This herb is sometimes used to bring on labor or to increase uterine contractions.

Comfrey root

Used topically for bruises, swelling, and pain relief, this herb is sometimes suggested to counteract the soreness of episiotomies and tears.

Slippery elm

Golden seal

Comfrey root

These are sometimes suggested for use in the bath to promote healing of an episiotomy or tear. The combination of all three is said to improve circulation and prevent infection as well.

Herbal preparations are not cure-alls and should be used with care and prudence, under guidance from your caregiver. The main problem with herbal remedies is determining their safety. If they work, they must be potent. And if they are potent enough to effect changes in the cervix or digestion, are they safe? It is very difficult to know how much of an herb to take. We don't really know how to regulate these "natural" remedies.

5

Oh, My Aching Back, and Other Joys of Pregnancy

With pregnancy come some very common (and very annoying) discomforts. I've listened for years to a litany of complaints from thousands of pregnant women. Below you'll find midwife-approved, mother-tested methods of solving—or living with—these problems plus some information on moods and lifestyle concerns that women frequently ask me about.

But first take a look at the following list, which shows some of the changes your body goes through from month to month. With the dramatic adjustments your body must make, it's little wonder that discomforts occur.

1 month: After conception, your progesterone and estrogen levels rise and you miss a period. You may already feel "different." The uterus is expanding, the cervix is becoming softer. Breasts can be tender as they grow larger, your pelvis may ache, and nausea can begin. Vaginal secretions may increase and you may feel faint.

2–3 months: As the embryo begins to form and the placenta is completed, your breasts become fuller; nausea and fatigue escalate or continue. The fetus's brain and nervous system are beginning to develop. You have to urinate more frequently. You may suffer mood swings due to the hormonal changes in the body.

4 months: Amniotic fluid increases and the placenta is busy providing nutritional, respiratory, and excretional functions for the fetus. Fetal movement may now be noticeable. Nausea usually disappears but constipation may now be a problem as intestinal muscles become sluggish.

5–6 months: The placenta is full-size and contains two to three pints of amniotic fluid. Joints are starting to relax in preparation for childbirth. Blood volume is way up and may cause gums and nose to bleed. Weight gain increases at the rate of about one pound per week.

7 months: The uterus has grown even larger. You feel more focused on the baby and delivery. You may develop backaches, heartburn, hemorrhoids, and varicose veins.

8 months: The uterus is just below the breastbone. There is little room left for anything else. Blood volume increases 30 to 40 percent. The heart enlarges and must pump about ten beats per minute faster than usual to accommodate the needs of your little passenger. Your ankles may swell, stretch marks appear, perspiration and urination increase.

9 months: The head is engaged, the cervix begins to efface. You experience Braxton-Hicks contractions and signs of imminent labor begin.

The complaints, discomforts, and pregnancy-related topics below are listed alphabetically so you can quickly flip to the issue that concerns *you* most.

Back Pain

AFFECTS YOU MOST: Months 5, 6, 7, 8, 9

Pelvic joints loosen during pregnancy, in preparation for the flexibility needed at delivery time. The loose joints, combined with the heavy load you're carrying, throw your body off balance and may cause low-back ache.

WHAT TO DO:

1. Try the pelvic rock: Get down on your hands and knees. Arch your back like an angry cat, then bend it the opposite way so that it flexes. Don't move your head or shoulders.
2. Learn to stand properly, with pelvis tucked. Here's how to get the hang of it: Place your feet at shoulders' width and tuck your buttocks under (this is the right way to walk and stand). To get an exaggerated feel of how *not* to walk and stand, arch your back slightly and push your hips to the front and buttocks to the back.
3. Try to avoid standing for long periods. Rather than stand for an hour making dinner, try to do some preparation in the morning and some of the work in the evening. Sit down to peel vegetables.
4. When standing for any length of time, try elevating one foot on a low stool to relieve back pain.
5. Don't wear very high heels. Choose shoes with good support. Try going barefoot.
6. Be careful when lifting. Bend at the knees, not at the waist, and lift with your legs, not your back.
7. Be careful not to gain too much weight. The added weight means more strain on your back.
8. Take warm baths to soothe tired back muscles or try using a heating pad.

Bleeding Gums

AFFECT YOU MOST: Anytime during pregnancy

Gums often bleed when you brush your teeth during pregnancy. This doesn't mean you have gum disease. It is simply the result of increased blood volume.

WHAT TO DO:
1. Keep your teeth clean and healthy.
2. Use a softer toothbrush.
3. Go to your dentist during pregnancy to have your teeth cleaned.

Braxton-Hicks Contractions

AFFECT YOU MOST: Months 8, 9

Although the uterus will contract starting at about the sixteenth week of pregnancy, these contractions are not regular or painful and are rarely felt by the pregnant woman until the eighth month. They are called Braxton-Hicks contractions and produce no change in the cervix the way true labor contractions do. Women pregnant with their second or third babies (these women are known as multiparas, or multips) feel these contractions sooner and more frequently than first timers (primagravidas). In fact, late in a multip's pregnancy, Braxton-Hicks contractions may get regular, occurring every five minutes or so, and can become more powerful each week.

WHAT TO DO:
1. Learn to distinguish between Braxton-Hicks contractions and labor contractions. Real labor builds and doesn't stop. Braxton-Hicks contractions may seem stronger this week than last week, but they will not get stronger or longer as the hours pass. In fact, if you change your activity (sit up, lie down, walk), they go away. Real labor contractions do not go away, no matter where you roam (and believe me, I've seen many

a mother-to-be try to escape them)! See Chapter 6 for more on real versus false labor.

2. If you're still not sure if this is real labor and you're concerned, call your doctor or midwife, even if your due date is far off. It may be premature labor. Premature delivery can often be prevented if premature labor is caught in time. A vaginal exam will determine whether the contractions are real labor, as your cervix will be changing in response to them.

Breast Soreness

AFFECTS YOU MOST: Months 1, 2, 3

Tender breasts are often the first sign of pregnancy. The soreness is due to increased levels of the hormone estrogen. You will also notice that your breasts grow in size. Some women like this; others hate it. The nipples darken and you may get stretch marks. Small bumps on the areolae (known as Montgomery glands) appear. Both the tenderness and the growth rate should subside after the first three months. By sixteen weeks, colostrum, the precursor of breast milk, may be present and can sometimes be expressed from the nipples. Some women will leak colostrum even late in the pregnancy. Other women couldn't express anything if they were to try. The colostrum is in there, though.

WHAT TO DO:

1. If breasts are so painfully sensitive that even gentle touching hurts, be sure your partner knows this. The sensitivity should decrease by the middle months and this aspect of your sex life can return to normal.

2. If your breasts are heavy, wearing a bra will be more comfortable than going without one. Be sure to buy some new bras one or two sizes larger than your regular ones to fit your new shape.

3. In the last month, you may want to prepare your nipples for breast-feeding. This isn't mandatory; your nipples will survive breast-feeding even without any extra assistance. Preparation

may, however, prevent some of the soreness that accompanies those first few days with your baby. To prepare nipples for the vigors of breast-feeding, you can try rubbing your nipples with a towel, sunning topless for a few minutes each day, or going braless for a couple of hours a day (so that the nipples rub against your clothing).

Dreams (Scary Ones)

AFFECT YOU MOST: Months 7, 8, 9

Most women report having scary dreams during pregnancy. Usually these dreams are about the labor or about whether the baby will be normal. Dreams also frequently revolve around what an incompetent mother you will be! (Fathers have dreams and nightmares like these, too, but they usually don't talk about them.) It helps to know that these dreams are normal, even common. Think of them as a way of working through problems that are so threatening they can't be dealt with consciously.

WHAT TO DO:
1. Talk about your dreams with someone else. Talking will help you to understand your own conflicts and concerns and may help you to deal with them realistically.
2. Look on the bright side. There may be a connection between women who have scary dreams and faster labors. These women have already worked through many of the conflicts and are more at peace with the idea of parenthood.

Edema (Swelling)

AFFECTS YOU MOST: Months 7, 8, 9

Mild swelling of the hands and ankles is a normal result of an increase in body fluids during pregnancy. You may notice more swelling late in the day or in warm weather.

WHAT TO DO:

1. Elevate your feet when you sit or lie down.
2. Lie on your left side.
3. Increase the amount of water you drink to help flush out your system.
4. Seek help for sudden or unusual swelling. Swelling can occasionally be the indicator of a more serious problem, such as preeclampsia or eclampsia, more commonly known as toxemia, and also called pregnancy-induced hypertension, or PIH. See Chapter 3 for more information on PIH.

Exhaustion

AFFECTS YOU MOST: Months 1, 2, 3, 8, 9

In the early months of pregnancy, you may feel like someone has sapped all the energy right out of you. The smallest tasks can seem overwhelming—you'd really rather just stay on the couch with your feet up, thank you. This flulike feeling is very upsetting to women who are used to being on the go. If you have other children to care for, the exhaustion will loom even larger. You may assume that if you feel this rotten now, you'll only feel worse later. Happily, this is not the case. The tired, draggy feeling will, like a heavy fog, simply lift one day (around the end of the third month or beginning of the fourth) and you'll feel bright and alive again. The final month or two of pregnancy can also be tiring because of the added weight you move around with, but even this tiredness cannot compete with the total exhaustion and lethargy you may feel in those early months.

The fatigue women experience during the first trimester is due to the pregnancy hormones that are at work making a life-support system for your baby. At the moment, your body is diverting all its extra energy to the task of nurturing this fetus.

Unfortunately, husbands do not always understand why their wives are acting like zombies when there aren't any visible signs of the pregnancy yet. You look okay to them, so they assume you should act normal, too. And because most women still carry the heavier load around the house, husbands often act irritated when meals aren't made and dust and laundry are piling up in the house. Ask your partner for help with specific chores. Most men will rise to the occasion if approached in a positive way. Once men understand that the exhaustion is due to hormones and is not an emotional or relationship problem, they can act appropriately.

WHAT TO DO:
1. Go to bed earlier. Get up later.
2. Take naps.
3. Get some exercise. This improves your circulation and gets needed oxygen to all parts of your body.
4. Find out from your doctor or midwife if you have anemia. You may need to take extra iron.
5. If you can afford it, hire someone to come and clean your house once a week or every other week. If you can't afford this, simply cut back on household chores and learn to live with less perfection for a few months.
6. Try to get a friend or baby-sitter to take care of your other children a few days a week.
7. If you are working, find a quiet place to go during your lunch hour—a couch in a coworker's office where you can close the door and relax would be ideal.
8. Make sure your diet is nutritional and balanced. See Chapter 4.
9. Get some fresh air.
10. Don't overschedule your days—you just can't do as much right now as you used to do. Say no to social outings, extra work, and volunteer work if you don't feel up to it.

Feeling Faint

AFFECTS YOU MOST: Months 1, 2, 3, 4

During early pregnancy, do you ever feel as if you are going to pass out? Seeing black spots before your eyes and fainting is not uncommon in the early months. Medical experts believe this occurs due to the effects of estrogen on a woman's body. The estrogen causes the veins and arteries to expand early in pregnancy in order to accommodate the increased blood volume (up 50 percent) that will be circulating through your body by twenty-eight weeks of gestation. If a pregnant woman stands or sits for a long time, the blood in her legs begins to pool due to the enlarged vessels and enlarged uterus, preventing the easy return of blood back to heart and head. Women who stand waiting for a bus, for instance, may begin to feel faint because of the decreased amount of blood returning to the brain.

WHAT TO DO:

1. Heed the early warning signs of fainting (racing heart, sweating, nausea, and seeing black for a few seconds). Sit down or lie down and let the blood return to your brain before you try to get up again.
2. Don't sit for prolonged periods without moving around or blood will pool and cause you to faint when you try to stand up.

Feeling Hot

AFFECTS YOU MOST: Anytime during pregnancy

Have you noticed that you are always hotter than your partner when you sleep now? It's very common and very normal to feel overheated. A pregnant woman's resting body temperature is elevated.

WHAT TO DO:

1. This is not a problem that needs treatment. Just keep in mind that a higher body temperature is normal and wear light sleepwear to bed; put the blanket on your partner's side of the bed only.

Fetal Movement

AFFECTS YOU MOST: Months 4, 5, 6, 7, 8, 9

Almost every mother-to-be worries: Is the baby moving often enough? Is the baby moving too much? Although the fetus begins moving by seven weeks, most pregnant women don't notice any movement until the sixteenth to the twentieth week. Fetal movement feels like a flutter. Often it's low in the abdomen, right above the pubic bone. Second-time mothers often feel the baby move sooner than first-time mothers, as early as sixteen weeks, because their abdominal muscle tone is more relaxed and they know what fetal movement feels like. Often this translates into a woman believing that her second baby moves more than the first.

Of course, some babies *do* move a lot more than others. Some mothers are more aware of the activity of the fetus than others. Most babies seem to have a pattern of movement over each twenty-four-hour period. They are often quiet, probably sleeping, as the mother moves about during the day. When the mother is moving, the baby is being rocked in the cradle of her uterus. When she lies down to rest, this often wakes the baby up (look out—babies do the same thing *after* birth!). The pattern of movement babies keep in the womb may have some effect on how they respond after birth. For example, most babies fuss and cry between 5:00 P.M. and 10:00 P.M. every night. Perhaps they're simply used to being rocked at this time. When they were in the womb, this was when the mother was quite active: returning home from work, making dinner, and putting other children to bed.

Sometimes you may notice repeated rhythmic kicks and you'll wonder what on earth the baby is doing. He's hiccuping! Babies in the uterus often get hiccups—this is normal. There's no need to try to find a way to stop them; babies don't seem to mind them.

A number of women report a fetal movement that feels like the baby is having a convulsion. The baby seems to startle and tremble all over; then movement subsides. I experienced this in one of my pregnancies and it *is* alarming, but it seems to have no relation to the baby's health or development. One theory is that the fetus is experiencing a movement known as the Moro reflex within the womb. The Moro reflex is a healthy sign in a newborn. It occurs when the baby is startled by a sudden loud sound or feels he or she has lost balance. The body stiffens and arches, arms and legs thrust outward, as though the baby wants to grab on to something.

Another fetal movement you may experience: late in pregnancy some babies turn themselves from head-first to foot-first (breech) or vice-versa. This intrauterine somersault feels like the baby is kicking and moving his arms and legs all over at the same time. When the baby quiets down again, you may notice you are being kicked in a different place. A head-first baby will kick you under the ribs. A breech baby will kick you in the bladder, rectum, or vagina; it may even feel like a foot will drop out. (It won't!)

WHAT TO DO:

1. Some caregivers ask women to chart fetal movement in order to assess the baby's well-being. This is one noninvasive method of measuring your baby's well-being before birth. The system involves recording the amount of time it takes before the first ten movements of the day occur. Patients are instructed to record the hour they wake up, then count ten movements and write down the time of the last one. Kick charts may make some women feel less anxious about fetal health. If you feel fewer than ten fetal movements by 2:00 P.M., sit down for an hour and pay attention to them. If you still do not feel at least ten movements, contact your physician or midwife. There is a correlation between a dramatic decrease in fetal movement and fetal stress and even death.

2. If you note a sudden and unusual decline in movement over a twenty-four-hour period, see your caregiver. The baby can be given a stress test to assess his or her health.

Fitness Concerns

AFFECT YOU MOST: Anytime during pregnancy

Exercise during pregnancy benefits mother and baby. Exercise keeps your weight down, increases blood circulation, and gives you a good feeling. It will even send you into labor better able to cope with the physical challenge of childbirth. The question is, how much can you do safely? And which sports are the best during pregnancy? These issues are still being debated by the medical community, and studies are under way to find the answers to our questions. Here's the best advice based on what we currently do know.

WHAT TO DO:

1. If you are out of shape and have not been exercising, join a pregnancy exercise class. These classes include stretching and very mild conditioning exercises.
2. Pay attention to your body's signals. If you feel faint or weak, or if you get a muscle cramp, stop exercising. Next time, do less.
3. Don't push yourself. Competitive sports are better left until after the birth.
4. If you're too tired or queasy to exercise during the first trimester, accept it. Don't try to force yourself. Don't feel guilty about being a couch potato for now.
5. When exercising, always make sure that you follow up with plenty of fluids, especially in the summer. You don't want to get dehydrated.
6. Do not use saunas or hot tubs. The temperatures are too high. The fetus cannot eliminate the heat the way you do.
7. Try bicycling, swimming, walking. Swimming builds muscle tone, improves circulation, and increases endurance. As you become larger, swimming has the added benefit of making you feel weightless!
8. Remember that your sense of balance is not what it once was. Sports like ice skating, roller skating, and ballet are fine to pursue if you are used to them, but your center of gravity

is changing with your growing belly. Beware of slips and falls that may result from this new balance. If you do fall, don't worry about the baby. A tumble rarely causes complications because the fetus is so well protected and insulated by your body and the amniotic sac. If you suffer an unusually strong impact to the abdomen, however, see a physician. A very strong blow can sometimes cause problems.

9. If you have been jogging prior to the pregnancy, you may continue to do so during the pregnancy, as long as you are experiencing no pregnancy-related problems. Make sure you stretch well before setting out and keep the pace *slow*. Don't overdo.

10. Do not begin a new sport or suddenly become an exercise fanatic if you used to lead a sedentary life. Do sports in moderation and use common sense. Refer specific questions to your practitioner.

Heartburn

AFFECTS YOU MOST: Months 5, 6, 7, 8, 9

Heartburn is a burning feeling in your chest and throat. It is the result of acid in the stomach being brought up. Your digestion is working more slowly these days. Also, the pregnancy hormones cause the valve at the top of the stomach, which usually keeps food and acids down, to soften. Late in pregnancy, heartburn may be caused by the pressure of the uterus on the digestive organs.

WHAT TO DO:
1. Eat early in the evening.
2. Sip milk. Some women swear by this.
3. Dry crackers work well for others.
4. If you notice that some foods aggravate your heartburn, avoid them.
5. Eat smaller meals.
6. Chew slowly and well.

7. Avoid greasy foods and fried foods.
8. Reduce, stop, or change iron supplements. These can some-times make heartburn worse. Ask your practitioner to rec-ommend a coated iron supplement, which may reduce irritation.
9. Sleep propped up in bed. See the section on sleep difficul-ties, page 116.
10. Ask your practitioner about using Tums.

Hemorrhoids

AFFECT YOU MOST: Months 6, 7, 8, 9

Hemorrhoids are a bulging of the wall of the rectum through the anal sphincter muscle. If you suffered from hemorrhoids before pregnancy, they'll probably worsen as your pregnancy progresses. They may occur due to the increased weight of the baby, uterus, and placenta. Hemorrhoids feel huge but are usu-ally the size of a marble or smaller. They hurt and burn and may bleed after a bowel movement.

WHAT TO DO:
1. Get a topical medication like Preparation H to help shrink the swelling.
2. Lubricate your finger with Preparation H and push the hem-orrhoid back in. Then tightly pull in the pelvic floor muscles. (See pages 167–168 to learn how to locate your pelvic floor muscles.)
3. Next, lie down and elevate your hips on a pillow for ten or fifteen minutes. This will help reduce the size of the hem-orrhoids, although it won't make them disappear perma-nently.
4. Avoid constipation because it can make hemorrhoids worse. Drink eight glasses of water a day. Eat whole-grain breads and cereals and eat lots of raw vegetables. Walk a mile a day. The exercise is good for your digestion.
5. Remember, although hemorrhoids can get worse during the

actual birth, they do improve after delivery. You will be much better within weeks after childbirth.

Inverted Nipples

AFFECT YOU MOST: Anytime during pregnancy

Some women worry about their possible inability to breast-feed due to inverted nipples. Although your breasts will produce the same amount of milk, inverted nipples are hard for the baby to latch on to.

WHAT TO DO:

1. Prepare nipples for breast-feeding by gently drawing them out with your fingers.
2. Gentle sucking can work just as well, if you and your partner feel comfortable with this approach.
3. Woolrich shields can be worn inside your bra. These help to coax out inverted nipples.
4. Inverted nipples sometimes begin to change by themselves as you get closer to the birth.

Leg Cramps

AFFECT YOU MOST: Anytime during pregnancy

A lot of women get terrible cramps in their calves or feet. Sometimes leg cramps awaken them in the middle of the night. It's thought that the cramps are caused by a calcium/phosphorus imbalance.

WHAT TO DO:

1. To prevent cramps, take more calcium in the form of calcium tablets. More milk won't work as well because it raises the levels of both calcium and phosphorus. Get calcium gluconate or calcium lactate (you don't need a prescription) and take

two or three 300-mg tablets per day. It's easy, it's cheap, and it works. Ask your practitioner about it.

Nasal Congestion and Nosebleeds

AFFECT YOU MOST: Months 4, 5, 6, 7, 8, 9

Because of increased blood volume, your nose may become stuffy. Some women also have nosebleeds, as the vessels near the surface are subject to irritation. Nasal congestion is quite common and can be an annoyance. It may get worse as you get closer to term. The congestion and nosebleeds may also increase in the winter months when you are subjected to dry heat indoors.

WHAT TO DO:
1. Don't use medications or nasal sprays.
2. Drink six to eight glasses of water a day.
3. Use a humidifier in the winter to counteract the dry air. Be sure to clean the humidifier and put in fresh water daily.
4. Blow your nose gently, so as not to cause a nosebleed.

Nausea and Vomiting

AFFECT YOU MOST: Months 1, 2, 3, 4

At least 50 percent of women experience nausea and vomiting in early pregnancy due to hormone changes. These symptoms may be present anytime during the day but are most common in the early morning and late evening.

WHAT TO DO:
1. Read pages 82–84 in Chapter 4 for ideas on how to combat nausea.
2. If you are vomiting more than once a day and are losing weight, contact your doctor or midwife for advice.
3. If you are vomiting constantly, stop drinking and eating every-

thing to break the cycle. Sometimes your stomach lining becomes so irritated that nothing will stay down. Call your doctor or midwife right away. You can lose a lot of fluids with constant vomiting. It might be better to spend a night in the hospital with an IV and observation than to risk dehydration.

4. Severe vomiting may not be pregnancy-related. After the first trimester has passed, food poisoning would be suspected. If you are in the care of a midwife, she may consult with her backup physician.

Pigmentation Changes

AFFECT YOU MOST: Months 4, 5, 6, 7, 8, 9

Pigmentation changes can include: (1) A dark line up the abdomen from the pubic bone to the sternum, which means nothing and will fade after pregnancy. (2) Mask of pregnancy, characterized by brown patches on the forehead and cheekbones. Again, nothing to worry about. This, too, will fade away after the baby is born. (3) Darkening of the nipples and areolae. This is perfectly common. Your normal coloring will return after birth.

WHAT TO DO:

1. For mask of pregnancy, be sure to stay out of the sun or use sun block when you are outside. The sun can make the patches worse.

Pubic Bone Pain

AFFECTS YOU MOST: Months 7, 8, 9

The bones of the pelvis can start to ache if you stay in one position for too long. Sometimes, when you swim or run, they can rub together and hurt. Mine hurt so much during one of my pregnancies, it felt like my pubic bone was broken. (Don't worry, it wasn't . . . and yours won't break either.) This happens because during pregnancy estrogen works to soften the cartilage in the middle of the pubic bone.

WHAT TO DO:
1. Talk with your caregiver about taking Tylenol for the pain.
2. If too much movement is the culprit, decrease your walking, swimming, or stair climbing.
3. Wait—delivery is the only real cure.

Round Ligament Pain

AFFECTS YOU MOST: Anytime during pregnancy

Some women get a sharp pain on either side of the uterus when they stand up quickly. The pain can also occur when urinating or when turning over in bed. This is known as round ligament pain and is usually nothing to worry about. It is a normal part of pregnancy. The round ligaments support the uterus in the pelvis. They start at the top of the uterus (the fundus) and end at the pubic bone. As the uterus grows, the ligaments stretch. They tend to cramp easily when you change position suddenly and you may get a sharp, momentary pain on one or both sides of the uterus. The pain disappears within seconds.

WHAT TO DO:
1. Try not to make any fast moves. Get up slowly and turn over in bed carefully, so you don't pull these ligaments.
2. If the pain does not resolve itself in a minute or less, or if the pain persists, it may be the sign of something more serious than round ligament pain. Persistent pain may be caused by a urinary tract infection, appendicitis, or—if it occurs in the first twelve weeks of pregnancy—a tubal (ectopic) pregnancy. Call your health-care provider.

Sciatic Nerve Pain

AFFECTS YOU MOST: Months 6, 7, 8, 9

The main symptom of sciatic nerve irritation is a pain that travels diagonally across the buttocks and down the back of the leg. The sciatic nerve often becomes irritated during pregnancy. The pelvic bones are loosened at the joints due to high estrogen levels, giving the pelvis more flexibility during the labor. This is beneficial during labor, but during pregnancy can irritate the sciatic nerve and produce mild to severe pain. The problem is aggravated by prolonged standing, stooping, and lifting, as well as by wearing shoes that give poor support.

WHAT TO DO:
1. Wear good running shoes or go barefoot.
2. Apply ice to the area that hurts: back of the hip or on buttocks.
3. Try a heating pad if ice doesn't help.
4. When you sit, put your feet up on a stool so your back doesn't arch.
5. Get up from your chair and move around every hour or so.

Sexual Issues

AFFECT YOU MOST: Anytime during pregnancy

What happens during pregnancy to a woman's sexual desire? Anything! Some women desire sex much more frequently, while others notice no change, and still others notice a decrease in sexual interest. There is no right or wrong way to feel. Equally often, the change in sexual activity is due to the man's feelings about the pregnancy. He may have mixed feelings about your new figure or worry about the possibility of sexual intercourse hurting the baby. Humans are complex creatures and something as monumental as expecting a baby is bound to change your sex life in some way. If you had a good sex life before conception, however, pregnancy should not dramatically alter it. In the same vein, if you had any sexual problems before the pregnancy, these will usually continue or sometimes become more severe during pregnancy.

Sexual interest may change *during* the pregnancy as well; you and your partner may feel more sexy some months than others. For example, if the first trimester is marred by fatigue, nausea, and vomiting, it is unlikely that your sex life will flourish at this time.

In the second trimester, things will probably return to normal or even get better. Some women find that pregnancy's increased blood flow to the pelvic area heightens their sexual interest and satisfaction. Their partners may also find the engorged genitalia more pleasurable, as it can make for a tighter fit. On the other hand, since vaginal secretions increase during pregnancy (more so for some women than others), the opposite effect can sometimes occur—the vagina may feel too loose and slippery for the man.

During the last trimester, the size of the woman's ever-expanding abdomen seems to provide a challenge for some couples and may interfere with lovemaking. Psychological changes at this time can also play a role in altering sexual feelings. The couple, each in his or her own way, are worrying about the birth and adjusting to the idea of parenthood. No longer does the couple see themselves as a pair of lovers. They begin to see themselves instead as mother and father, a concept that obviously changes the nature of the marital relationship either in a very positive way or sometimes in a negative way. Because the woman's size makes the baby seem so much more "real," some couples feel as though there are now three people in bed instead of two. This feeling of being "spied on" by the baby makes some couples uncomfortable. Nervousness about hurting the baby through sex may also increase at this time.

WHAT TO DO:

1. Keep in mind that intercourse is perfectly safe during all of pregnancy until the membranes rupture. The only exception

to this rule is if there has been bleeding or threatened prematurity.

2. Let your partner know that sex cannot hurt the baby, who is very well protected within the amniotic sac. The mucus plug also keeps the baby safely sealed away, and there is no danger of infection from sex at this time. Furthermore, a normal pregnancy will not be thrown into early labor by sexual excitement.

3. For comfort, you may have to try different positions to accommodate your growing middle. The standard missionary position will become less and less comfortable as the pregnancy continues—you'll want your partner's weight off your abdomen.

4. The only sexual practice that is not safe is blowing air into the vagina. This can cause an air embolism to enter the bloodsteam and is extremely dangerous.

5. Talk with each other about your feelings about sex, your needs and concerns and desires.

6. Talk also about issues unrelated to sex but that may affect your sex life. For example, worries about your ability to be a good parent, fear of the approaching labor and delivery, concern over your attractiveness, anger over being the one who has to do "all the work" of pregnancy, etc. If these issues aren't aired outside the bedroom, they're likely to crop up in your sex life.

7. If you're having trouble working things out, tell your health-care provider. We have heard it all and nothing is going to shock or embarrass us. Often a third, neutral party can be a help. Your health-care provider may suggest that you see a counselor. This can be a positive experience for couples learning to deal with all the stresses of family life.

8. Remember that your changing emotions and changing feelings about sex are normal. All expectant parents go through some of these same things.

9. Don't use the frequency of sex as a way to measure your love for one another. It's possible that frequency of sex will decrease due to first-trimester nausea, feelings of fatigue,

third-trimester discomforts, or medical warnings during a high-risk pregnancy.

10. If your caregiver cautions against sex, find out the reasons. Ask specifically what is meant: no intercourse? no orgasm? no masturbation? If you had a brush with premature labor but got past it, find out if and when you can resume sexual relations or whether you are advised to abstain for the duration of the pregnancy.

Sleep Difficulties

AFFECT YOU MOST: Months 7, 8, 9

Sleeping in late pregnancy can be difficult at best and impossible at worst. The combination of your size, heartburn, breathlessness, leg cramps, and frequency of urination makes it a wonder pregnant women can sleep at all. Just turning over can be a monumental effort, and it may be hard for you to find a comfortable position.

WHAT TO DO:

1. Exercise every day, preferably out-of-doors, and you'll sleep more soundly at night.
2. Eat your evening meal earlier. This way you're not trying to sleep on a full stomach, and heartburn will be less likely to keep you awake.
3. Use extra pillows. Some women sleep best on their sides with a pillow under the head, another between the knees, plus a third supporting the abdomen and/or upper arm. Turning over, of course, becomes very complicated with this arrangement.
4. Some women have found that sleeping in a semisitting position works well for them. They use a large bed pillow with arms plus a few extra pillows for the head and behind the back. It's also good to get another pillow under the knees for support. This position can also be comfortable for labor.

Stretch Marks

AFFECT YOU MOST: Months 7, 8, 9

Stretch marks are dark red or purplish marks that occur when the skin is stretched beyond its capacity. They most commonly appear on the breasts, abdomen, and thighs. Some women don't get any (I don't like these women either!) and some get covered with stretch marks, which is unfair and undeserved.

WHAT TO DO:

1. If I knew the answer, I'd be a rich woman! There are a hundred-plus remedies (creams, lotions, massage) that claim to prevent stretch marks. The reason there are so many is because none of them works!
2. Avoid full-length mirrors late in pregnancy. A combination of stretch marks, weight gain, and pigmentation changes can make anyone have second thoughts about motherhood!
3. Look to the future. By three or four months after the birth, stretch marks will fade to a silvery color and be much less noticeable.

Unwanted Advice

AFFECTS YOU MOST: Anytime during pregnancy

One of the minor discomforts of pregnancy is the feeling that you have somehow become public property. Everyone around you thinks they have the right to ask personal questions and offer advice you never sought. You may also have to listen to unsolicited pregnancy horror stories. Many pregnant women find themselves in conflict with their mothers, mothers-in-law, close family members, or even friends during this time. The conflicts arise around a wide variety of issues, running the gamut from whether to use a doctor or midwife, where to deliver, what's safe, whether anesthesia is appropriate during labor to breast-feeding versus bottle-feeding, having children present at the birth, etc.

WHAT TO DO:

1. Let your mother and others say what they want to say. Don't argue or criticize, just listen. You may want to add, "I appreciate your concern" or "I'll think about it."
2. Don't let the pregnancy horror stories worry you. Some women just love to make birth sound worse than it is. If something someone told you is bothering you, mention it to your doctor or midwife, who should be of help in easing your fears or concerns.
3. If people make a remark like "You're too big" or "You're too small," discuss it with your caregiver. I am asked about this issue so often! Once you understand the wide range of normal pregnancy sizes, you'll feel less anxious.
4. Take all the advice and comments as a compliment. People care.
5. Remember, just because someone asks you a question doesn't mean you have to answer. If questions and comments seem too personal, just ignore them.

Urine Leaking

AFFECTS YOU MOST: Months 7, 8, 9

Here's a problem you seldom hear anyone talk about but that affects many pregnant women, especially those who've had children before. It is called stress incontinence. The urine may leak out when you laugh, sneeze, cough, or while vomiting. This is fairly common, although embarrassing. (If you could spend a few days listening to what women complain about in my office, you'd hear *everything* . . . and realize how normal you are.)

WHAT TO DO:

1. To keep anxiety levels down when you're in public, wear a minipad.
2. Strengthen and tighten the pelvic floor muscles, which hold in the urine, by doing the Kegel exercise. (See pages 167–168 for instructions on how to do a Kegel.) You'll want to start

doing twenty to thirty Kegels a day. This seems like a lot, but they're not hard to do and can be done anywhere. You don't need to set aside any special time for doing them. Your symptoms should improve within a few weeks.

Vaginal Discharge

AFFECTS YOU MOST: Months 4, 5, 6, 7, 8, 9

Increased vaginal discharge is a normal part of pregnancy. The discharge is thin and milky and may increase as you get closer to term. Sometimes it can be difficult to tell the difference between normal discharge and a vaginal infection. If you experience itchiness, burning and/or redness, or if there is a foul odor or change in the consistency or color of the discharge, an infection is probably the cause and you should see your midwife or doctor.

WHAT TO DO:
1. Keep the genital area clean and dry.
2. Wear cotton underwear.
3. Do not douche (unless specifically instructed to by your practitioner).
4. After going to the bathroom, remember to wipe from front to back, not back to front.
5. Avoid refined sugars. A poor diet can make you a more likely candidate for an infection.
6. Wear a minipad if this makes you feel more comfortable.
7. See your caregiver if an infection is suspected. Refer back to Chapter 3 for more information on some common vaginal infections.

Varicose Veins

AFFECT YOU MOST: Months 4, 5, 6, 7, 8, 9

The job of the veins is to return blood to the heart. They depend on a series of one-way valves to keep blood from backing up. Sometimes during pregnancy, the valves become weakened and blood backs up and pools. This puts pressure on the veins and causes them to bulge. Varicose veins are more common in women who have already had one pregnancy and in obese women. They also tend to be hereditary. The weight of the pregnant uterus and the increased blood volume put the pregnant woman at greater risk of varicosities. Varicose veins can occur in the legs as well as the vulva, vagina, and perineum.

Varicose veins bulge and ache when you sit or stand for long periods of time. Besides being uncomfortable and unattractive, they can be dangerous. They predispose women to blood clots in the area where the vein has popped out. Blood clots are dangerous because they can come loose and travel, perhaps lodging in the heart, lung, or brain.

Varicose veins of the vulva may look like they will interfere with a delivery, but they do not.

WHAT TO DO:

1. Wear maternity support hose. Put them on before getting out of bed in the morning. If you wait until you're up and about, the blood will have already had a chance to pool. Depending on the severity of your problem, there are a number of different kinds of hose with varying amounts of support. Check with your midwife or doctor on which to choose. If varicose veins run in your family, start wearing support hose *before* they happen to you. This way, you may be able to prevent them.

2. For varicose veins of the vulva, vagina, or perineum, try a folded sanitary pad in your underpants. This can apply some pressure on the vein and relieve the achiness you feel when you have to stand for long periods.

3. Get exercise! Walking, cycling, and swimming are best because they build up muscle tone in your legs, which will help pump the blood out. The exercise and improved circulation will help varicose veins of the vulva as well as the legs.

4. Lie down several times a day. Elevate your feet to drain blood from legs and vulva.

5. Avoid long stretches of sitting. Get up every hour and move around for five minutes or so before sitting down again.
6. Call your CNM or MD if you experience redness, painful swelling, and increased heat in any of your veins. This could be a sign of a clot forming and needs medical attention.

Work Stress

AFFECTS YOU MOST: Anytime during pregnancy

If you are healthy and work isn't too stressful (mentally or physically), you can work right up to labor. Working throughout pregnancy does not suit all women, however. You should not feel pressured to remain at work in the final months if you would prefer not to be there. Although many women *need* to continue work for the money, others are working because they feel they shouldn't ask for special treatment and worry that they will appear to be the "weaker sex." The superwoman image—of someone who can handle work, competition, travel, stress, and mother-hood as easily as baking a pie—is somewhat unrealistic. This is a very complicated issue for career women. I have counseled many tearful women in my office who are torn between their loyalties to their jobs and their soon-to-be-born babies. Fathers rarely even consider this issue and almost never wonder whether they should slacken the pace of their jobs for the sake of fa-therhood. A few women seem perfectly comfortable with the idea of working and mothering and manage to approach both tasks without feeling stressed or guilty.

WHAT TO DO:
1. Try to reassess honestly what you want from life in the next few years.
2. Don't buy into the superwoman dream. "Doing it all" is not for everyone. You have a right to consider other options, make other decisions without feeling pressure to be all things to all people.
3. Don't compare yourself to your husband and his abilities to

continue on at work. He does not physically experience the pregnancy; he doesn't give birth; he won't be the one nursing this baby. You have just undergone an amazing physical and emotional feat that, even if he has witnessed it, he can barely be expected to understand.

4. Look into options that may be more realistic for you. A large number of women opt for part-time work during their pregnancies or after the birth. If heavy lifting is involved on the job, a woman might want to ask to be assigned a slightly different job within the same organization during the pregnancy.

5. Whatever you decide to do, don't let guilt get in your way. You can be a great mother and still continue to work. If you decide to do this, you will not be alone in your decision. More than half of all women with children under the age of six are working today. Recent studies indicate that the children of these working mothers are bright, sociable, and independent. One study even found that children of working mothers have higher IQs, and another reported that they had higher reading scores. So remind yourself that you are not hurting your child by working.

6. Look back at your own childhood. If your mother worked, talk with her about how she coped. If she didn't work, your anxiety may result from your break with this role model.

7. Look at the bright side: your children will grow up knowing that a wide range of possibilities exists for them; their careers and parenting choices, we hope, will not feel so limited or cause as much angst as ours do.

8. Look at the workplace as something that can enhance family life, not compete with it.

9. Remember, when you feel happy, your baby will feel happy. So make the decision that's right for you, for your family, regardless of what today's trends and norms are.

Worrying That Something Is Wrong with the Baby

AFFECTS YOU MOST: Anytime during pregnancy

At some time during the pregnancy you may become convinced that something is wrong with the baby. Almost everyone feels this way. Statistically, however, you have every chance of carrying a healthy baby. If you've already had one normal birth, your chances of a healthy second baby are even greater. If you have had a previous pregnancy that ended in miscarriage, prematurity, a stillborn baby, or a baby born with a birth defect, however, your fears will be magnified, although not necessarily justified. Depending on the problem, it may be highly unlikely that such an event will be repeated.

WHAT TO DO:

1. Tell your midwife or doctor about your fears. Often he or she will have good evidence that your fears are unfounded.
2. Go for a sonogram. You'll be able to "see" for yourself that everything looks right. Amniocentesis may be an option as well. See pages 60–62 for more on the pros and cons of both these procedures.
3. Remember that statistically you have an excellent chance of having a normal, healthy baby. Only 3 percent of babies born in the United States have major genetic diseases. Unless you have been told otherwise by your caregiver, you have no reason to assume that anything should be wrong with the baby.
4. Life is a risky business, and pregnancy and parenthood make us realize how vulnerable we really are. No amount of testing, planning, and worrying can *guarantee* a perfect baby for any of us. After taking reasonable precautions, one needs to let go and trust. This is a lesson that all parents must learn and that is part of being a parent throughout life.
5. If you have had a previous baby born with a birth defect, you may want to seek genetic counseling.
6. If your last baby was delivered prematurely, you are at risk for another premature birth and will want to take precautions.

You may want to see a high-risk specialist. Ask your practitioner to explain all the signs of early labor to you so you can seek help quickly this time.

7. Talk with your spouse about your fears. Although no one really knows how he or she will cope with a child born with a birth defect or with the death of a baby, it is a good idea for you and your husband to at least get a few thoughts on this subject out into the open. For many women, especially those who know someone who had a baby with a problem, these fears can run quite deep. Although it's difficult to discuss pregnancy loss or birth defects while you are pregnant, it can help to face up to your fears. You'll sleep better at night.

Once you make peace with the many minor discomforts and major changes of pregnancy, you'll be ready to look forward to the work ahead: your labor and delivery. In the coming chapters, I cover everything you ever wanted to know about childbirth.

6

Dealing with Labor: Better Ways

As your pregnancy draws to an end, you will become more and more interested in, and concerned about, the labor and birth of your baby. You may have a lot of fears and worries. Many women wonder whether they'll be able to cope with the pain of labor and delivery. All women want to know what labor and delivery entail, what lies ahead for them. Although each labor is different (just listen to a few women talk and you'll hear how different), all labors represent the body's efforts to push the baby out into the world. Let's take a look at this miraculous process . . . and take the fear out of it.

For an unknown reason, sometime in the ninth month your body begins to produce a hormone called oxytocin, which causes the muscles of your uterus to contract and sends you into labor. The contractions are involuntary and you have no real control over them. They are also intermittent, never continuous, so there is always a rest in between contractions. This allows the woman time to prepare for the next contraction and gives the uterus and the fetus a rest as well. The frequency and strength of each contraction vary and depend on the stage of labor a woman is in. (See the section on pages 131–134 on the three stages of labor.)

The muscles work in two ways. In the early part of labor they work to pull the neck of the cervix up. Once this job has been completed (meaning that the cervix is fully dilated), the muscles work to push the baby down and out of the body. Their last job is to push out the placenta after the baby's birth.

Signs of Impending Labor

LIGHTENING

The baby's head drops down and engages in the pelvis. This often occurs about one to two weeks before labor for the first baby and often not until labor for subsequent births. The mother-to-be will notice that she has more upper abdominal room to eat and breathe but will feel greater pelvic pressure. This pressure can be uncomfortable. It may be coupled with leg cramps, due to the pressure of the head (or other presenting part) on the nerves of the legs. Swelling and varicosities can grow worse as well, since it is now harder for blood to return from the lower extremities. You will also notice more pressure on your bladder and greater frequency of urination. At last your long wait for the birth of your baby is almost over. A few weeks before your due date, take time to review—with your coach and caregiver—your plans for labor and the ways you would prefer your delivery to be handled.

CERVICAL CHANGES

Your doctor or midwife will probably do a vaginal exam during one of your last visits. By feeling with two fingers, your caregiver can determine whether the cervix (deep inside the vagina) is hard or soft, thin or thick, closed or open. You may be told that your cervix has begun to efface. This means that the cervix feels much softer to the touch and shorter in length. The neck of the cervix is beginning to thin. You will also be told if you have begun to dilate (that the cervix is opening). The changes in your cervix are probably due to the increased intensity of the Braxton-Hicks contractions. Although this can be exciting news, it does not mean that you are about to go into labor at any minute. The birth of your baby can still be weeks away. Be assured, though, that your body *is* getting ready for labor and the time for delivery is drawing near.

INCREASED BRAXTON-HICKS CONTRACTIONS

Your abdomen will feel suddenly hard and will painlessly or painfully contract. You have actually been having these contractions since about sixteen weeks' gestation, but they were previously unnoticed. Braxton-Hicks contractions are erratic and do not, like real labor contractions, escalate in frequency or strength. (See the section on false versus real labor on page 129.)

PREMATURE RUPTURE OF THE MEMBRANES

Sometimes (about 12 percent of the time), the bag of waters breaks before labor starts. This is what the baby has been floating in up until now. You will probably go into labor within twenty-four hours of this rupture. Contact your doctor or midwife to let him or her know what has happened. You will be instructed not to take a tub bath, douche, or have intercourse now that the waters have broken.

Amniotic fluid is usually clear (though it may be tinged with blood from the cervix), and some white flecks may be visible. These are fragments of vernix caseosa, a cheesy coating that protects the baby's skin as it floats in the amniotic fluid. If the fluid is dark with a brown, green, or yellow color, the baby has passed meconium (had a bowel movement), which indicates that there may have been some distress or that the baby is now in distress. Either way, the baby should be evaluated.

Occasionally, the waters leak instead of gushing out, and it can be hard to tell whether the leakage is amniotic fluid or urinary incontinence. You will have to check with your doctor or midwife as it is important to know if it was amniotic fluid.

PROLAPSED CORD

On rare occasions, the cord may wash down with the amniotic fluid. This is an emergency situation, for oxygen is being cut off to the baby. Call an ambulance. While you wait, get on your hands and knees with your head down and your bottom up. This position helps to get the baby's head off the cord and lets more oxygen through. When the ambulance or rescue squad arrives, ask for oxygen to breathe to help the baby as much as possible. When you arrive at the hospital, an emergency C-section will be performed.

BLOODY SHOW

A mucus "plug" has been guarding the entrance to your cervix during pregnancy. A couple of days to a week before labor, a small quantity of bloodstained mucus is expelled. This is called "show." It may appear off and on until labor begins and continue through the first stage.

EXTRA ENERGY

Many women notice a sudden spurt of energy in the final days before labor starts. This has also been referred to as the "nesting instinct," as you may find yourself suddenly busy with last-minute domestic preparations in anticipation of the baby. Although it's terrific to feel this sudden sense of vigor, do not overdo. Take it easy or you'll head into labor exhausted from overzealous housecleaning efforts.

DIARRHEA AND INDIGESTION

In the twenty-four to forty-eight hours preceding labor, a woman may have loose stools or mild diarrhea. This is quite common and helps to make room for the baby's head in the pelvis.

False Labor Versus Real Labor

The easiest rule of thumb to remember is that false labor will stop, real labor won't. So try to make it go away. Take a warm bath, a nap, get in a comfortable reclining chair with lots of support, and see what happens. If it continues, get up and walk around. If it is in the middle of the night, go back to sleep. No baby will be born with contractions that are twenty minutes or more apart, so ignore them. No baby has ever been born while the mother was asleep (you should be so lucky), so get some shut-eye. Don't sit up all night timing the contractions and getting worn out. If serious labor starts you'll be exhausted, and exhaustion is one of the enemies of a successful labor. If your membranes break, however, this is not false labor and you should report it immediately to your caregiver.

I would like to add one thing about "false" labor: there is nothing "false" about the mild pain you feel. That is real and uncomfortable. Furthermore, false labor indicates that real labor is just around the corner. So the use of the term "false labor" is somewhat of a misnomer. Perhaps it should be called "prelabor."

Baby's Position

The most common position (and the easiest to deliver) is with the baby's head down (*vertex position*) and chin tucked to the chest. Most babies get into this position by the seventh month. Unfortunately, not all babies oblige. Some babies in the vertex position do not tuck their chins to their chest and instead hold the chin up, military fashion. This makes the head a larger diameter to come through the pelvis and causes a more difficult delivery for the mother. Other head-down babies are facing the "wrong" way: with limbs to the front and spine to the back (posterior), as opposed to limbs toward the mother's back and spine to her front (anterior). Most posterior-position babies rotate by themselves at delivery. If not, forceps are sometimes used at the delivery to rotate the baby.

Other babies do not get into the head-down position at all. Some are in the *transverse position*, lying across the uterus with head on one side and feet on the other. A baby in the transverse position is always delivered by cesarean because he or she cannot get out sideways. If you wait until labor starts before you plan on a C-section, you may be happily surprised to find that the baby in the transverse position turns head-first just before labor starts.

A number of babies are positioned bottom-down in the *breech position*. There are basically three types of breech presentations: complete (the baby looks like he's sitting with legs tucked); frank (the baby makes a V-shape, with bottom down and legs extended straight up in front); and footling (one foot or knee dangles down and is the presenting part). The frank breech is most common. Breech babies are often delivered by cesarean because there is a risk that once the feet and body are out, the head (which is the biggest part) may get stuck. Some doctors will deliver a breech baby vaginally if the woman is a multip and the baby is in the frank or complete breech position.

Before actually engaging in your pelvis, the fetus is still free to move and somersault about. If a baby engages in the bottom-down position, there are a few things you and your practitioner can try to do to get him or her to turn. There is always the chance, however, that the baby will decide to turn back into the breech position (some babies fit better or are more comfortable in the bottom-down position).

To coach a breech to a vertex before labor starts: Lie on your back with your head on the floor and your bottom up in the air. To make this angle more comfortable, use pillows, furniture, or even a slanted ironing board to keep hips elevated well above shoulders. Remain this way for about ten to twenty minutes. Ideally, the baby will tip free of the pelvis and begin to move into a head-down position. You may feel the baby somersault. Afterward, have someone help you to get up, as you may be dizzy. Don't lie down right away or the baby may simply return to a breech position. Walk around, hoping that the baby will become fixed in your pelvis in the head-down position. The baby may not turn the first time you do this. Try the position twice a day for ten to twenty minutes each time, beginning in the thirty-fourth week of pregnancy, and continue for a month. Most babies will eventually turn. Sometimes your doctor or midwife can turn the baby manually through pressure on the abdomen, but there are risks to this procedure (such as pinching off the cord), and it is usually done in a hospital.

The Stages of Labor

In the *first stage of labor*, the neck of the cervix flattens out and widens enough to allow the baby's head to pass through. Once it reaches this point, you are ten centimeters dilated, or fully dilated. The *second stage* begins with the urge to push and ends with the delivery of the baby. In the *third stage*, the placenta is delivered. *Fourth stage* is described as the first hour following delivery of the baby. (Mothers and babies are carefully observed during the first hours after delivery, because if either of them is going to have complications, it is likely to happen then.) For the first-time mother, the stages of labor will probably go something like this:

2–6 hours   *Early Labor, First Stage.* Dilated 0–4 cm. Mild contractions of short duration (20–60 seconds) every 5 minutes. (In the very beginning of labor, the contractions will be more infrequent or irregular, possibly coming every 20 to 30 minutes and lasting 15 to 20 seconds.) Mild to moderate cramping in the lower abdomen, thighs, and lower back. Between contractions, the mother feels fine.

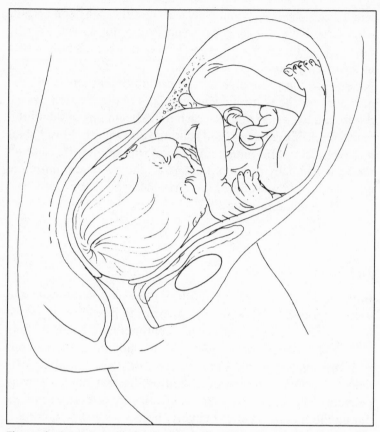

The mother's cervix is dilating (opening). The baby will begin its descent down the birth canal (vagina) once dilation is complete.

3–4 hours   *Active Labor, First Stage.* Dilated 4–7 cm. The woman feels moderate to strong contractions lasting 60 to 90 seconds every 3 to 4 minutes. As dilation approaches 7 cm, the labor becomes much more difficult and the woman may feel she wants to go home and forget the whole thing.

1–2 hours   *Transition.* Dilated 7–10 cm. The contractions are strong (60–90-second duration) every 2 to 3 minutes. As 10 cm

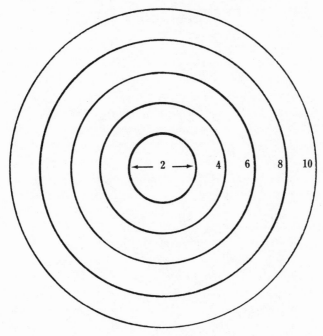

Dilation of the cervix is measured in centimeters. The cervix is fully dilated at 10 centimeters.

approaches, the contractions may get even closer to-gether. The woman can feel overwhelmed, panicky, and trapped. If membranes haven't yet ruptured, they are likely to do so now. Once you are at 10 cm, you are basically ready to push.

1–2 hours *Second Stage.* The contractions are farther apart again. They come every 3 minutes or so and last 60 to 90 seconds. These contractions should give the mother the automatic urge to push. She feels differently now— often a little happier and better able to communicate with others. This stage ends with the delivery of the baby.

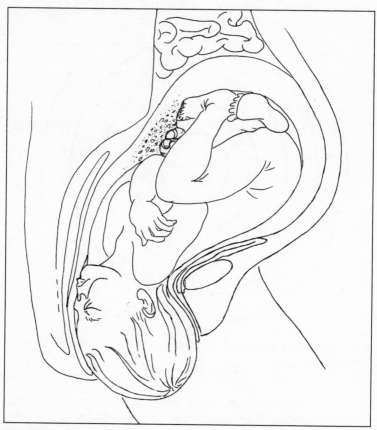

The baby's head is crowning. Your practitioner and coach can now see the top of the baby's head. This is a good time to look in a mirror so you can have the same encouraging sight.

5 minutes to   *Third Stage.* The baby is out and often still attached
30 minutes   to the placenta by the umbilical cord. The mother is
                asked to push two or three more times with the final
                contractions to deliver the placenta.

When to Go to the Hospital or Birth Center

It's better not to get to the hospital or birth center too early. Many more women arrive too early than too late. Going to the hospital won't make your baby come any faster. (The atmosphere there just isn't that relaxing.) And unless you're very nervous about being away from the hospital, you'll probably labor much more effectively at home in comfortable surroundings. First babies take twelve hours, on average, so you have plenty of time to get to the hospital without having to spend all day there.

How can you tell when to head to the hospital or birth center? It can be difficult to know with your first baby. You know how your contractions feel right now, but you don't know how much more intense they will become. To make matters more confusing, not all women follow a traditional textbook pattern of labor, with contractions progressing smoothly from ten minutes apart to five to three. Some women experience a long space between some contractions, then only a few minutes before the next one. Keep your eye on the longest space between contractions instead of the shortest. If you can still go ten minutes without a contraction, you're not in danger of delivering right this minute. It's best to wait until all your contractions are coming every four to five minutes, lasting sixty seconds, and strong enough to make you grimace. This probably means you're about four centimeters dilated. You will not be fully dilated until you reach ten centimeters. If your water breaks, you will want to call your caregiver right away.

If you get to the hospital and you're only one or two centimeters dilated, ask to go home until labor gets more serious. If you're in the labor suite too long in early labor, chances are greater that someone will decide to speed you up, that something may be wrong with your labor, when what's wrong is that you're there too early and should be at home!

Here's one woman's account of this early, iffy stage of labor: "My contractions began in the late Saturday night hours between 1:00 and 2:00 A.M. Instead of staying up to count the minutes and limiting my food and fluid intake, I went back to sleep. . . . The contractions intensified throughout the next day and I contacted the Maternity Center around lunchtime when they were about five to seven minutes apart. The midwife called me back and we decided that since my water hadn't broken and there was no show, to take a nap or a shower and call when things speeded up. Around four o'clock the contractions were getting harder to manage and I was feeling irritable. After consulting with the midwife again, we decided to come to the center."

Here, a four-time mother relates her story (yes, even after three previous births, it's still hard to know exactly when to head for your birthing location):

"My water broke at 8:25 the night of the thirtieth. Since this had happened on my previous birth and contractions last time had started within a half hour, I expected the same this time. I called the Maternity Center and spoke with my midwife. Being the calm person she is, she said, 'Well, call me when something happens.' I said, 'Fine.' Well, after all the rushing around and getting kids off to the baby-sitter, the contractions didn't start until 3:00 A.M. the thirty-first, but they were one minute apart! I immediately called [the midwife] and she said, 'Don't rush. I'll meet you at the center at 3:30.' I said, '3:30??!! How about 3:15?' . . . We packed into the car and proceeded down the highway at an alarmingly fast pace. I asked Frank to slow down . . . he must have been nervous because, despite my pleading, the speedometer read 80 mph. . . ." They met the midwife there and had their baby soon after.

How to Handle Early Labor

At first, your labor may seem fun and exciting. In the beginning, the contractions are not usually too strong and most women are excited that, at last, the baby is about to be born. What does a contraction feel like? It feels like a strong menstrual cramp, and its strength will increase throughout labor. Many women call me during this very early phase and they laugh and chat easily. Their contractions may be coming every two or three minutes, according to their calculations, but during a five-minute phone call they never pause. They sound like they've just won the lottery! (Even my husband now recognizes this as early labor and *he's* an architect!) During this stage, the best thing to do is to relax. Your body is just beginning its work. The cervix is effacing (thinning out) and you have time for a walk, bath (if waters haven't broken), or nap.

As early labor progresses, the contractions begin to last longer and they're much stronger (okay, for ninety-eight percent of us, they *hurt*). This is when you might start to get scared. This feeling of panic is temporary. You will soon get used to this next, more powerful stage, known as active labor.

How to Handle Latent Labor

Latent labor is, essentially, an extended early-labor phase that does not progress to active labor. Sometimes a woman continues to have contractions that, although bothersome enough to prevent sleep and cause pain, do not dilate the cervix. These contractions may not be particularly painful, but they can have a demoralizing effect on the woman, who soon realizes that she just isn't getting anywhere. The worst part of latent labor is exhaustion.

Whether this labor should be pushed along or slowed down is often a dilemma. Sometimes sedatives are given to suppress nonproductive labor. They don't work very well, however. Other times, labor is hastened by rupturing the membranes, stretching the cervix manually, or giving an enema. This often doesn't work well either. The best thing to do is to try to deal with the labor until it becomes more productive on its own. I advise a woman experiencing a very long early-labor stage to sleep, take warm baths (if the membranes haven't ruptured), and eat and drink high-carbohydrate foods (toast with honey, graham crackers, juice). The coach needs to offer support, understanding, and patience for the woman's mental health. This is a difficult stage of labor to pass through calmly.

How to Handle Active Labor

As you move into active labor, think positively about the pain. *These* are the contractions that will really move you along in labor. They are much more productive than those you experienced during the first two to six hours of early labor. During this stage you need to work *with* the contractions, not against them. Concentrate on "letting go," giving in to the power of the labor. Just as you were taught to relax your limbs in childbirth classes by talking to them ("Relax your shoulders, relax your arms . . ."), I believe that you should talk to your cervix during labor. It may sound strange, but it works just as well as the relaxation exercises you have practiced. Think to yourself, "Let the baby out, let the cervix open, open up inside . . . let the baby come down." Imagine a circle getting bigger. These are also helpful statements for your coach to make in a low, sure, and calm voice.

Here are some tips for coping with the pain of active labor:

1. Stand in the shower during labor. This is warm and relaxing. Besides, standing up helps the labor to progress.
2. Sit in the Jacuzzi, if it's available. We have one at the birth center and many women make it through those last few centimeters in there. In the Jacuzzi you feel weightless, and the waters do wonders for calming the anxiety of labor. We jokingly call it the Birth Center epidural because of the good pain relief it affords.
3. Breathe deeply, in and out. Don't hold your breath during a contraction. Your coach should breathe with you.
4. Relax between contractions. Your coach should remind you to do this and point out any tense areas. If the coach simply places his hands on an area of your body, this should be your cue to relax and release the muscle tension there. He should also watch for frowning or clenched teeth and encourage you to let the jaw relax, let the forehead relax. It's important for your coach to remind you where the tension is.
5. Get into any position that is comfortable for you: kneeling, on hands and knees, standing with arms around coach.

6. Stay upright as long as possible. Continue to walk around.
7. Keep the lights in the room dim.
8. Play soft music.
9. Remind yourself that this is pain with power and purpose: it is bringing your baby closer to you. Try to welcome the next contraction, not fight it.
10. A little ice applied to the lower back along with massage may ease the pain of back labor. Or a heating pad may be right for you.
11. A hot-water bottle placed over your lower abdomen may be comforting.
12. Try talking to yourself, repeating simple, optimistic phrases like "My baby will soon be born" or "My cervix is dilating."
13. The coach can help you to relax by giving massages in between contractions. Usually a light touch works. The coach should do whatever feels best for the mother. He can work on the shoulders, arms, legs, back, and abdomen. Sometimes, just lightly stroking these areas helps the woman relax better. The coach should use lots of praise such as "That's good. Rest in between."

Here are excerpts from some letters written by women who gave birth at the Maternity Center. They talk about how they handled the pain:

- "The pain was awful. Back labor was never one of my strong points. I can deal with regular labor quite well, but honestly, it felt as though someone was bashing my lower back with a baseball bat. I had to use my deepest concentration to control the pain. After going back and forth to the bathroom and the bed, I finally got the urge to push. . . . I said, 'My back is really hurting.' Suddenly I heard the wonderful words of encouragement from my midwife: 'Kim, if you push, the pain will go away.' Of course, I pushed and pushed—and you know what, the pain did go away!"
- "Laboring at the Maternity Center was a calm, quick (three and one-half hours), and sometimes humorous period, due

in a large way to the relaxed and experienced assistance of
our midwife . . . and her attendant . . . (an hour under the
pulsating shower head helped, too)."

- "A strong dose of common sense and compassion instead
of the popular, highly overrated drugs of the hospital is all
that is needed for the birth experience."

- "I didn't want to be touched, or anyone to even get close
to me. I had to work it out on my own with total uninter-
rupted concentration, and with the breathing and relaxation
I was doing just fine."

- "Having found that swimming pools and bathtubs were the
best places to be comfortable through the last weeks of
pregnancy, I got in the Jacuzzi during my labor, *sans* bubbles
for me. It did a wonderful job of helping me relax through
and between contractions. But the best help in relaxing
came from my wonderful husband, who climbed into bed
with me, holding me, and gently encouraged me through
what proved to be a long labor."

- "At one point, I started saying, 'Noooo, I can't do this'
during the contractions. . . . The midwife told me to say,
'Yessss, I want this baby to come out,' a psychological boost
that surely did more for me than a 'boost' of drugs. It certainly did it more gently, and helped build my confidence
for the next phase."

Labor: How Long Is Too Long?

Although each woman is different and no set time limit should
be rigidly imposed on the length of a labor, there are times when
a labor goes on too long and puts mother and/or baby at risk.

The lengths of women's labors can vary widely. I have seen
normal births take as little as thirty minutes or as long as forty-
eight hours. As a rule of thumb, a woman's second labor is about
half the time of her first. Length of labor and its safety for mother
and baby are hotly debated issues. Medical research has been
extensive, and yet no hard-and-fast rules can be applied to all

labors. Many factors need to be considered when evaluating how long is too long to spend in labor.

Safety is, of course, the prime issue. The mother's safety is relatively easy to assess (we can see her, run tests on her, talk to her), but the baby's safety is harder to gauge. Even with our very best technology, we have limited access to the baby before birth and it can be hard to assess how well the baby is tolerating labor. The fetal heart tones are the most commonly used method to predict fetal distress or well-being. In some cases, fetal scalp sampling (which is done only in certain hospitals) can be used to get more information on the well-being of the baby. A small scrape is made on the fetal scalp in order to collect a sample of blood, which can then be analyzed for oxygen and carbon dioxide levels. If the baby appears fine and there is every reason to believe that he or she will remain fine for the next few hours, then labor can be safely allowed to continue. The mother's health must be looked at carefully as well. Any signs of infection, exhaustion, or high blood pressure might indicate that she has been in labor too long. How effective her contractions are is also a clue as to whether or not the labor is normal.

I also try to determine what might be causing a problem labor. At this point I would look at a few things.

First, is the mother a small woman with an apparently large baby (over nine pounds)? If so, there might be a problem with the baby's ability to fit through the mother's pelvis. This is known as cephalo-pelvic disproportion (CPD). If the CPD is not severe, the problem resolves itself, as the baby's head molds to fit the shape of the pelvis.

Possibly, the baby is not in a good position. Perhaps his or her head is extended rather than flexed, making it more difficult to negotiate the pelvis in the expected amount of time. If the baby's heartbeat and all other parameters of a normal delivery are found, waiting just a little bit longer sometimes does the trick.

There may be an emotional reason behind the slowdown rather than a physical one. A woman may suddenly stop making progress in labor because she is tense and is fighting her labor. This can cause the cervix to stop dilating. If relaxation methods, coaching, warm baths, and different positions don't help to relieve her anxiety, a small amount of Demerol or, if the delivery is being done in a hospital, an epidural can be administered to help her to relax.

When labor slows or stops, the reasons behind this turn of events and the safe options must be considered. Obviously, there is always the option of the C-section available to resolve the problem of a prolonged labor. Watchful waiting and less invasive methods should be tried in the meantime. Rupture of the membranes, for example, or Pitocin, which can be administered in the hospital, usually work to get better contractions going before a C-section needs to be considered.

Induction of Labor

Labor can be induced mechanically by midwives and doctors before your body spontaneously begins the process. Why are inductions done? Usually labor is induced to ensure maternal or fetal health. If the pregnant woman has worsening high blood pressure (also known as eclampsia or PIH, pregnancy-induced hypertension), the woman should be delivered as soon as possible. Induction can also be used for pregnant diabetic women. Or if labors preceding this one were so fast as to jeopardize the mother's safe attendance by a doctor or midwife in the hospital, in the birth center, or at home, then induction might be considered. Fetal indications for induction include *intrauterine growth retardation* (sometimes the baby is not being well-nourished by the placenta and it may be better for the baby to continue growing outside the womb at this point); an *overdue baby* (there is still some controversy about how late is late); *premature rupture of membranes* (if no labor begins after the membranes rupture, the woman is usually induced before twenty-four hours have passed because the baby is at risk for infection and the longer you wait, the more serious the risk becomes); *moderate to severe Rh disease*. In this disease, an Rh-negative mother builds up antibodies against an Rh-positive baby. Her first Rh-positive baby would be fine, but a second pregnancy with an Rh-positive baby causes buildup of antibodies. The mother's system may actually attack the baby's red blood cells. The baby is at risk for developing severe anemia, jaundice, and even brain damage. This disease, however, has almost been eliminated with the advent of the drug RhoGAM, which prevents the mother's body from producing the antibodies. Within seventy-two hours after the birth of the Rh-negative mother's first child, she is given RhoGAM if the baby is Rh-positive. Because there is always the chance the baby's red blood cells have crossed to the mother during pregnancy, many practitioners advise taking RhoGAM during the first twenty-eight weeks of pregnancy and again seventy-two hours after the baby's birth if the baby turns out to be Rh-positive.

The ways in which a woman can be induced vary greatly. To have a successful induction, the cervix needs to be soft and effaced and slightly dilated. If time permits, the cervix is sometimes softened with prostaglandins in preparation for induction. Prostaglandins are drugs in suppository form that can be inserted directly into the vagina, causing the cervix to soften, efface, and dilate before labor induction is begun.

Labor can be started either by relatively "natural" methods or by more mechanical means. Natural methods are numerous but don't always work. In one method, the examiner manually stretches the cervix with her fingers and then loosens the membranes that are stuck to it, which is known as stripping the membranes (their adherence to the cervix is loosened, but the membranes are not actually ruptured). Often, when the woman then gets up and walks around, productive labor is stimulated. The disadvantages to this method include some discomfort as the examiner stretches the cervix and loosens the membranes, the possibility that it will produce unproductive contractions, and the risk that the examiner may instead rupture the membranes. An enema can also be given to induce labor (it is theorized that labor contractions are set off by the irritated bowel). Another natural method, which may seem surprising to you, is nipple stimulation. When the nipples are massaged, oxytocin is naturally released into the mother's bloodstream, just as it is during labor.

The baby's heartbeat should be monitored carefully during this time. Intercourse can also sometimes stimulate labor in a woman who is ready to deliver. The woman's orgasm causes a big contraction, which may be enough to start her labor.

If no labor starts with these methods, more intrusive methods can be tried. The membranes can be ruptured. Once ruptured, labor often starts spontaneously. If it does not, however, there can be problems, as the baby's risk of infection increases as time passes. Labor can be induced with Pitocin, a synthetic oxytocin. The drug is very similar to what women naturally produce during labor. Pitocin is administered by IV and must be carefully regulated and discontinued abruptly if there are any signs of fetal distress. During Pitocin use, the baby's heart rate should be continually monitored to determine how the baby is responding to the contractions. The advantage of using Pitocin is that it is a powerful drug that will most likely work. In this same strength lies its disadvantage. Pitocin can cause hyperstimulation of the uterus and fetal distress. The contractions it produces are much more painful than nature's own and can be difficult for the woman to cope with. Furthermore, each woman's body responds differently to the drug, making it difficult to tell how much is needed.

Obviously, induction should be used only when the benefits outweigh the risks. It must be reserved for situations in which it is medically indicated and not done for the convenience of the mother, midwife, or physician.

Tips for Coaches

As the labor continues, coaches will want to keep these suggestions in mind:

- Stay close by. Do not move around without telling the mother where you are going. She depends on you.
- Hold her; don't wait until she feels she must grab you. Holding her reinforces comfort; letting her grab you produces panic.

- Tell her to concentrate on opening up and letting the baby out.
- Use simple reminders: "Relax your face, relax your shoulders, let the cervix open, see that circle inside getting bigger . . ."
- If you notice any tension, help her by talking her through it: "Let your body go soft and sink into the bed. Let your body get heavy and let the bed support you."
- Make eye contact.
- Keep calm and still.
- Encourage her to sleep between contractions if she can.
- The harder and more intense her labor gets, the quieter you have to keep the atmosphere.
- Don't make conversation. Keep sentences simple. Say "Have an ice chip" and leave it at that.
- Praise her for her efforts: "You're great." "That's perfect." "One contraction at a time." "You can do it." "Good work." "You're relaxing beautifully." "You look just like the woman we saw in the movie."

7

The Delivery, Made Easier

Giving birth is not a passive process. It is an active, very physical drive that compels a woman to push the baby forcefully out of her body. You are the main participant in your baby's birth. Think of yourself as the catalyst here. You cannot depend simply on being "delivered" by your caretaker. You can attend classes to better understand intellectually what happens, but with or without classes and books, women already know how to give birth, just as they know how to menstruate, conceive, and grow babies. Some women deliver with relative ease, but most struggle and sweat to get the job done and some need extra assistance to accomplish the process safely. There are no tests or grades. This is not a contest. It is a part of life.

Positions for Delivery

There are a number of different positions that a woman can assume for delivery—some will feel right to her, others won't. Unfortunately, a few may be imposed on her by hospital rules or a practitioner's preference.

146

ON YOUR BACK

Despite all that has been written about alternative delivery positions that seem to be preferable for the mother, the supine delivery position remains the most common, usually used by doctors in hospitals. Most often, the woman is on a delivery table, sometimes with her legs and feet up in stirrups. Although this angle provides the best view of the birth for the doctor, it has many disadvantages for the mother and baby. Blood flow to the baby is reduced because the uterus is pressing on a major blood vessel, the inferior vena cava. The mother is forced to work against gravity to push the baby out. With legs up in stirrups and difficulty pushing, there is a greater chance of tearing and/or episiotomy. If you had hoped to avoid an episiotomy, this position makes it very difficult to do so. The birth outlet cannot stretch gradually to accommodate the baby's head and is more likely to tear.

Although so commonly used, this is not a position a woman would ever naturally assume if left to her own devices. The only time I would suggest that a woman get flat on her back for a delivery is when the baby is in a head-first position but with the back of his head to the mother's back (occiput posterior) or head-first but with the head turned sideways (transverse head-first position). In these fetal positions, it is very difficult to get the baby under the pubic bone. The supine position will sometimes get the baby "unstuck" and under the pubic bone. The mother lies flat on her back with no pillow under her head and pulls her legs back, holding them in place with her hands under the back of her knees. She looks like she's about to do a backward somersault—it feels strange but is worth the effort because it works so often. This position makes more room in the back of the pelvis for the baby to come down. The change in the angle helps the baby to get under the pubic bone.

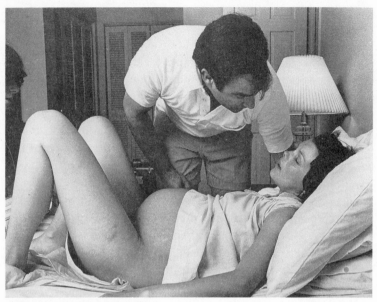

Waiting for the final contraction

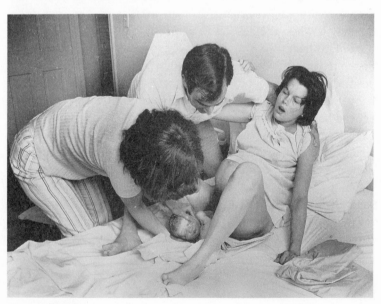

The head emerges

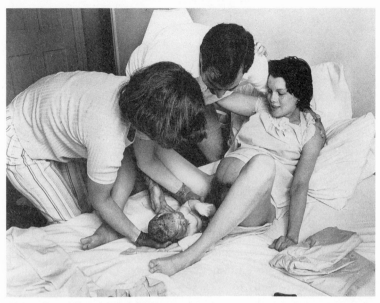

The mother's first smile of welcome

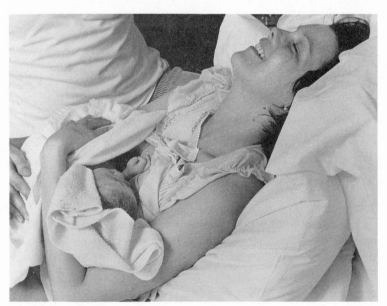

The miracle of birth

SEMISITTING

With the help of lots of pillows, a forty-five-degree angle can be achieved. Labor-room beds can often be adjusted to this angle for a comfortable semisitting position. Sitting up is a position that works with gravity to help you push the baby out. Blood supply to the baby is good because there is no extra pressure on the vena cava, a major vein. Most women at the Maternity Center deliver sitting up. It allows for good support and relaxation between contractions. Also, the coach can get behind the mother and help support her.

HANDS AND KNEES

This position works especially well for women with low-back pain. Once on hands and knees, push down toward your rectum. If this position seems to help you to push most effectively, use it. Most physicians have very little experience helping a woman deliver in this position and may feel uncomfortable with it.

LEFT LATERAL

The woman lies on her left side in a slightly fetal curl. The coach holds up her top leg to make room for the baby and then the woman pushes down toward her rectum. Although this position doesn't work with gravity (the way sitting/squatting positions do), it has the benefit of lessening tension around the birth outlet and reduces the chances of a tear or episiotomy.

SQUATTING

A laboring woman can safely squat on a bed. She should get on her feet with knees far apart, facing her coach. With arms around the coach's neck or shoulders, she is able to push down hard toward the rectum. Although this position can speed delivery considerably, it is hard to maintain for any long period. Squatting on the floor can be a little easier because you can stand up between contractions. If you end up delivering on the floor, your midwife has to be very flexible (literally) to see what's happening. I use a small mirror on the floor under the mother to see how fast the baby's head is coming. I also move all delivery equipment to the floor and cover the area with clean pads to receive the baby. It's not comfortable for the midwife, but if it gets the baby out, then that's what we do.

SUPPORTED SQUAT

The woman squats on the floor but is supported by a coach who holds her from behind, usually under the arms. She has the benefit of being in a vertical squatting position without having to support her own weight. She also has freedom of pelvic movement because she is not restricted to bed, chair, or stool.

BIRTHING STOOL

By using a birthing stool, a woman can sustain a squat position because she is supported. It is somewhat akin to sitting on the toilet, a place where many women instinctively feel most comfortable during labor. We associate this position with a bowel movement and the familiarity often frees a woman to use the same expulsive muscles to move the baby down and out. This position makes the second stage pass much more quickly. Your midwife may have a birthing stool and could arrange to have it at a hospital or home birth. Ask about this if you are interested. Doctors rarely have or use these stools.

BIRTHING CHAIR

The birthing chair has been installed in some hospitals but is often not used because it is "different." The chair helps to keep women upright, which speeds their labor and encourages effective pushing. Women also appreciate being able to see their caregiver, as opposed to having to stare at the ceiling when on a delivery table. Some women find the chair too rigid or uncomfortable. Once in the chair, you can't really move around. The use of squatting, birthing chairs, and stools during the pushing phase, however, may cause a little more swelling than other positions, as the blood pools and collects in vagina and labia. This causes no real harm, though, and it does get some "stuck" babies delivered!

Pushing Strategies

Pushing is a natural urge. Left to her own devices, a woman would instinctively know how to push her baby out. Occasionally a fully dilated woman does not feel the urge to push. This usually indicates that the baby has not descended far enough and is not yet pressing on the pelvic floor. On the other hand, some women feel the urge to push before they're fully dilated. This can be due to a baby whose head is very low in the pelvis. Although it's difficult not to respond to this urge, women must not push until they're fully dilated or they may cause the cervix to swell or tear. A few women seem to take a break after full dilation, and there is a short period of quiet (ten to fifteen minutes) before the need to push begins.

Once you're ready to push, certain techniques may be helpful to keep in mind, as they can help you to deliver with less effort. Be sure to wait for the urge to push and push *with* it. This helps you to push the right way. Pushing is most effective when it is timed with your natural contractions. Sometimes you won't have an urge to push, but usually you will. When you do get the urge, try putting your chin to your chest when you push. This dramatically increases your ability to push effectively. Tightly squeeze the abdominal muscles over the very top of the uterus. This added push from above can help get the baby out. Also, relax your jaw as you push. Open your mouth. Don't clench your teeth. An open mouth helps to open the vagina (it may sound strange, but it really works). Think about opening up, relaxing the perineum. If you don't make any progress within fifteen to twenty minutes (I don't mean delivery; I mean progress moving the baby down), then change position and try something new.

All women, especially first-time mothers, feel stuck while pushing. It feels like the baby will never fit. Then it feels like you will burst apart. Your initial reaction when the baby's head is crowning is to pull back, put your knees together, and get out of the hospital or birth center through any available exit! The pressure of the head makes you feel as though you'll be split in two, and you can't imagine how the head will fit through. Everyone feels this way. These are very scary sensations, but they indicate that you are very close to getting your baby out. The trick is to open up and let go, to *relax*. This can be the most rewarding part of labor.

Contrary to what you might have heard or read elsewhere, not all women like to push. Some women feel better pushing because they feel they are at last *doing* something. But about half of the women I see don't like pushing and would rather do almost anything else. You don't have to like it to do it well. Even if you hate pushing, it will be only an hour or two out of your lifetime and you can cope. Soon you'll be holding your baby.

Here's what one second-time mother had to say about the pushing phase: "When it came time to push, I was scared because with my first child I hadn't felt anything because of anesthesia. In my mind, I remembered the two hours of pushing with my first child, but little did I expect for this second baby to make an appearance in under ten minutes! My water had never broken throughout the labor and he was born with the bag still intact. The midwife told me this was called 'born in the caul' and traditionally meant that Brendan would be lucky and fortunate the rest of his life."

Another mother says she lost the urge to push: "I couldn't feel the contractions or the urge to push anymore so I waited and waited, probably about ten minutes. Then the midwife said, 'Well, you must be having contractions because I can see the baby's head going in and out . . . so why don't you just go ahead and push so we can have this baby!' Well, you didn't have to ask me twice. I pushed and pushed until suddenly out came the head, followed by the body—and for the unbelievable fourth time, we had yet another boy!"

A first-time mother describes the pushing stage this way: "We pushed for a long time—over three hours. This time was confusing for me though never hopeless. Pushing is like nothing I've ever felt before (analogies to bowel movements notwithstanding), and for all our practicing, it still felt otherworldly to me. We continued to try all the birthing positions from all the cultures all around the world, searching for the one that would work for us. The baby's heartbeat was still strong through all of this. Then an angel in the form of Marion McCartney appeared and said, 'Why not try squatting?' and, lo and behold, our baby came close to crowning. My husband held a mirror so I could see just how close we were to having our baby in our arms."

Time Limit on Pushing

Statistically, the first-time mother pushes for one to two hours. Subsequent babies take an hour or less (the majority take a half hour). These are not absolutes. A caregiver must judge the situation in order to decide when the pushing has gone on for too long. Perhaps the woman pushed ineffectively for the first hour and then got the hang of it in the second hour. She is still within a reasonable time limit then. My basic rule of thumb is that pushing can go on as long as progress is being made, there is no fetal distress, and the woman is not totally exhausted. I have seen mothers push for as long as three to four hours, but they progress and they do get these babies out on their own.

Many variables affect how quickly a woman will push her baby out. If a woman has had an epidural, her second stage may be considerably slower. This is because the drug takes away the natural urge to push. Often, low forceps are used to facilitate this delivery. Maternal exhaustion can be another real disadvantage in this stage because a tired mother cannot push effectively. Glucose, by mouth or by IV, can help to give her some needed energy for the second stage. Continued praise for her progress is also essential. If the mother's pelvis is small in relation to the size of the baby's head, this can make for a tight fit and the pushing stage can take longer than is ordinary. A side-turned (transverse) head or posterior head position can make it very difficult to push the baby out as well. If the strength and frequency of the contractions diminish substantially, the second stage will slow down and it may be necessary to take measures to augment the labor. Inadequate effort by the mothers due to inexperience or lack of good direction will inhibit effective pushing as well. It's a good idea for all first-time mothers to practice different positions, and to ask for direction from the staff wherever they deliver.

If things are not progressing, it sometimes helps to take a fifteen-minute break from pushing. During this time, I ask the woman what she fears most or dislikes most at this point. Often I find out she is afraid of tearing or feeling out of control, or she's afraid the baby will be born with birth defects. There are many fears pregnant women have at birth and expressing them often makes them more manageable. Once they've gotten their concerns out in the open, they're better able to push the baby out. The break, by itself, helps some women to regain their composure and suddenly gives them a better, clearer urge to push. You have time to pay attention to what your body is telling you.

It takes time, patience, goodwill, judgment, cooperation, and trust to help women deliver.

Delivery of the Placenta

Once the baby is out and breathing, you will probably forget all about the placenta. When the midwife or doctor reminds you to push this last bit out, you may groan. Don't worry. Placentas are very easy to deliver after birth. They have no hard or bony parts to hurt you. You simply push as the doctor or nurse-midwife puts gentle traction on the cord. Most placentas come out easily.

After that, the nurse or midwife will massage your uterus to keep it well contracted and to prevent excess blood loss. This "massage" may feel a bit rough to you. Sometimes it hurts, and you may wonder why you're being attacked. But there is a very good reason behind this massage. If the uterus stays firm and well contracted for the first two hours after birth, there is minimal blood loss and you will feel better. Ask for a demonstration so you can massage your uterus yourself.

If You Tear

Sometimes the woman tears unexpectedly, either in addition to an episiotomy or without one. It's not the end of the world if you tear. It can always be repaired, just as an episiotomy can be. (For details, see page 165.) You are not a failure because delivery is not a contest! Keep it in perspective. Nobody's delivery is perfect.

A Word About Underwater Births

I do not advocate underwater birth, even though some people believe this is easiest for mother and safe for the baby. I have been at many deliveries where the baby's breathing was mildly to moderately depressed at birth. On dry land, these babies are fairly easy to resuscitate, but I would be afraid of the added risk of having a baby aspirate water at delivery time before I could begin resuscitation efforts. Of course, laboring in the bath or Jacuzzi is fine and often very helpful for pain relief (see Chapter 6, page 138).

Tips for Having Children at the Birth

I have been at a number of births with children present. Most of these experiences were positive. Some were not. One four-year-old was absolutely thrilled with the event and bonded in a very immediate and positive way to the new baby. Another patient of mine wanted her two daughters, ages four and six, to attend the birth, but when she went into labor, they refused to leave the birthday party they were attending to see the birth. Obviously, the magician they were watching seemed more exciting to them than the idea of a sibling's birth. Most children have no concept of the birth itself and are fairly egocentric. I have, however, seen a child as young as four coach his mother through birth in a supportive and loving way. This was a child who had been born with congenital heart problems and had already been operated on two times. During labor, he sat with his mother's head in his lap and stroked her forehead and breathed with her. He really understood pain and knew what made it feel better. He had all the moves of an experienced coach. It's one of the few times I've seen a child act like an adult during labor.

Whether or not your children are actually present at the birth, they can still bond in a special way with the new baby. The most important ingredient in this bonding is your general attitude toward pregnancy, birth, and the newborn. If you seem open, honest, calm, and happy, your children will retain a positive feeling about pregnancy. And even if they're not there for the actual birth, you can probably arrange to have them there soon after delivery to hold and see the new baby. Here are some tips if you decide to go ahead and have children present during labor and delivery:

- Take them with you to a few prenatal visits. Let them listen to the baby's heartbeat and meet the person who will be delivering the baby.
- Bring them to the hospital or birth center if this is where you plan to deliver. Let them tour the labor and delivery rooms, see babies in the nursery.
- Prepare them beforehand by telling them a little bit about birth. Get them to share their feelings with you in advance. Do they want to be there? Are they looking forward to the new baby? Are they worried? Jealous?
- All children need a baby-sitter for the birth, one who will

explain what is happening in a language they understand. The sitter should know the children well and be sensitive to their needs.

- If a child wants to leave the birthing room, don't interfere. Respect his or her wishes. Never carry a child back into the birthing room.
- Use an open-door policy, allowing the children to come in and out as they wish.
- Don't expect them to appreciate the magnitude of the moment. Some kids just aren't all that impressed.
- Remember, a small child thinks the world centers on him or her, not you. Don't be surprised if he or she walks in during the delivery and asks you to make dinner.
- Your attitudes about the birth will be reflected in your child's behavior. If you have reservations about having your children at the birth, they will sense this. If you are frightened of childbirth or worried about how you will cope, they will pick up on this, too. Don't have children attend unless you feel very positive about this birth.

An eleven-year-old girl and seven-year-old boy who witnessed the birth of their new baby sister wrote to the Maternity Center with the help of their parents. Michael said: "It was exciting to watch her come out, but I didn't know it would look so messy. My favorite part of the whole thing was holding her right after she was born. It made me feel responsible for her. I thought her hair would be light like mine, but it's really dark." Monica said: "It was really neat to help with the birth of my new sister. I ran lots of errands for everybody and . . . I got to cut the umbilical cord after she was born. That makes me feel even more special and close to her. She's so tiny and cute and cuddly. I knew she'd be small but not as small as she actually is. She feels soft and comfortable in my arms."

Normal labor and birth can progress without intervention from medical personnel. As technology has improved, however, we have developed so many ways of helping women to move through labor and delivery that these "aids" are often used even when they are not medically necessary. In the next chapter, we will cover these interventions, explaining when their use is justified, why a normal birth may be better off without them, and give tips on how to avoid unnecessary intervention.

8

Your Baby, Your Way: Decisions About Childbirth

You have just read two chapters outlining normal labor and delivery. But not all childbirth experiences move along without a hitch. Some require medical assistance. Others may not require medical intervention, but the hospital staff or doctor may offer or suggest it. There are a number of birthing decisions facing every pregnant woman, decisions she will make with her midwife or doctor. This chapter will help you decide what's right for you.

Before you head into labor, you'll want to form a birth plan with your wish list of actions to avoid or try. Discuss your thoughts with your caregiver now: don't wait until you're in labor. If you haven't had a baby before, you may not be sure of what you want. At this point, you're probably very concerned about the possible pain of labor and the safety of birth for your child and yourself. The information below will help you decide what's best for you and show you how to avoid any unwanted interventions during a normal delivery. During your labor and birth, you'll want to avoid routines that undermine your confidence, are uncomfortable or hurt, or pose a threat to the likelihood of a normal delivery. A midwife is trained to assist you in reaching this goal. Should the situation change and warrant intervention, you must rely on your practitioner's medical advice.

Enemas

Nobody wants one and lots of women get one. Midwives do not use them routinely. Some physicians have also stopped using them routinely because they're so unpopular and often unnecessary. The thinking behind their routine use has been to empty the lower bowel to make more room for the baby's passage through the birth canal. The truth is that many women in early labor have diarrhea (nature's enema) and their bowels are already empty in anticipation of the birth.

WHEN YOU MAY NEED THIS PROCEDURE

If a woman has been constipated a day or two before she goes into labor, she may want an enema. Usually Fleet enemas are used; they are small and not too painful. Often, an enema *does* have the advantage of moving labor along to the next stage and can sometimes get contractions that have stopped started up again.

WHY YOU MIGHT NOT WANT THIS PROCEDURE

The enema is uncomfortable, often serves no useful purpose, and only upsets the laboring mother. She may feel that she is not being allowed to go through birth in a dignified manner.

HOW TO AVOID THIS PROCEDURE

If you're horrified by the thought of an enema, discuss it with your doctor or midwife. Avoid the routine by speaking up! If you have been constipated and agree that you need an enema, you can sometimes do it yourself at home *before* you're in hard labor, and in a place where you feel more private and comfortable. Many women are concerned that they will have a bowel movement while pushing and be embarrassed. I have seen bowel movements happen as women push, and some women aren't even aware of it. In the pushing stage, you will be concentrating on nothing but the birth; it is a very intense stage and it is unlikely that *anything* will embarrass you then anyway. If women express concern about it beforehand, I simply tell them that if they do have a bowel movement, it's no big deal. I just change the pad underneath them and go on. Furthermore, I let them know that having an enema is no guarantee a bowel movement won't happen.

Shaving

Happily, this routine has been on the decline in obstetrics. Shaving of the pubic hair was thought to keep the area cleaner for delivery and for repair of episiotomies and tears. I have never shaved any of my patients and find no greater incidence of infection. In fact, most of the medical community now agrees that there is a greater chance of infection from the nicks and scrapes of the razor.

WHEN YOU MAY NEED THIS PROCEDURE

If pubic hair is quite long, clipping it does make it easier to sew up tears or episiotomies, but shaving is not necessary.

WHY YOU MIGHT NOT WANT THIS PROCEDURE

Having your pubic hair shaved by a nurse is unpleasant and undignified. There is a chance of nicks, scrapes, and infection. As the hair grows back, your skin is itchy and irritated.

HOW TO AVOID THIS PROCEDURE

Again, you can probably avoid this routine by speaking up. If a shave is hospital policy, just be sure that you have something in writing from your doctor so that the labor nurses know your doctor has okayed your decision to skip the shave.

Episiotomies

This is a surgical cut made with scissors into the vagina and down toward the rectum to enlarge the opening for delivery. The incision is routine in the United States and is very difficult to avoid in most hospitals. I am always amazed at how many pregnant women have never heard of an episiotomy and how many more women never even discuss the issue with their caregivers. It is, sad to say, a surgical procedure that can be performed without consent. Most obstetricians advocate the episiotomy for a number of reasons so far unsubstantiated by medical literature. Like most midwives, I believe that the episiotomy has its place but should not be done routinely or without cause. Unfortunately, most doctors who routinely do episiotomies have no idea what would happen without one because they've so rarely seen or managed a normal delivery without cutting. In my practice, close to ninety percent of my patients do not need an episiotomy. These women are not extraordinary, and I am not a magician. But after fifteen years of avoiding the episiotomy, I do consider myself an expert on the subject. Obstetricians could easily learn how to avoid the episiotomy and avoid damage to the perineum as well.

If your midwife or doctor decides it is necessary to do an episiotomy, you should know that there are several variations on this one theme. Different practitioners cut differently. There is the midline episiotomy, which many consider the best, as the cut is in the same area as a natural tear would be (straight down from the vagina in the direction of the rectum). The midline cut seems to be more comfortable afterward and easier to repair. It has been likened to unraveling a seam in a fabric as opposed to cutting across the grain of the fabric with scissors. The other type of episiotomy is the mediolateral, which instead of going straight down the center of the perineum is cut diagonally to one side. The thinking behind this type of incision is that it will prevent a tear from continuing on to the rectum. The mediolateral is more difficult to repair than a midline and takes longer to heal. If you know beforehand that your doctor is likely to do an episiotomy, I would suggest talking about these various cuts and requesting that a midline episiotomy be performed. Of course, if forceps need to be used or if the caregiver thinks that in your particular case this type of cut would only extend, then the mediolateral may have to be made instead.

WHEN YOU MAY NEED THIS PROCEDURE

The episiotomy should be considered when:

- the baby is in distress and needs to be delivered quickly
- forceps need to be used
- a breech baby is being delivered vaginally
- a severe tear looks likely
- a small women is delivering a very large baby
- an unusually tight perineum seems unable to stretch any farther

WHY YOU MIGHT NOT WANT THIS PROCEDURE

I'm willing to wager that the majority of women would choose *not* to have an episiotomy if someone offered them a choice. And for very good reasons:

1. There is no evidence to support claims that childbirth by episiotomy is safer than giving birth without one.
2. There is no evidence to support claims that having an episiotomy preserves the pelvic floor muscles better than not having one.

3. Doctors claim that they use the episiotomy to avoid tears. Yet in the instances when women do tear, they rarely tear to the extent and length of a routine episiotomy.

4. Doctors say they do episiotomies to avoid a tear that could extend to the rectum. A recent study done at the University of California, San Francisco, and reported in the May 1989 issue of *Obstetrics and Gynecology* seems to indicate that just the opposite is true. In a study of 2,706 women, researchers found that those who were given midline episiotomies had rectal tears almost nine times more often than those who received no episiotomy. In fact, in their study, 90 percent of all reported rectal tearing occurred *with* the episiotomy. And, ninety-seven percent of women *without* episiotomies had *no* rectal damage.

5. If a tear should occur, it can be repaired with stitches in the same way as an episiotomy. A jagged tear is more difficult to sew than a straight surgical cut but is worth the effort because a tear heals more easily and hurts less. Like any other skill, of course, sewing a tear must be learned and practiced. But if I, as a CNM, have learned to do this, surely an obstetrician, for the sake of his or her patients, can as well!

6. Women tear much less frequently than they receive episiotomies. In the study of 2,600 births managed by midwives at a Bronx, New York, hospital and mentioned in Chapter 1, about half the women had intact perineums after birth. And, as I mentioned earlier, at the Maternity Center, close to 90 percent of delivering mothers have no episiotomies. Those who do tear rarely tear to the extent and size of a regular episiotomy. Their tears are easily repaired and heal well. So I really see no reason to cut an episiotomy routinely. It seems so much safer to deliver without one. Yet in many hospitals routine episiotomies are done more than 90 percent of the time, supposedly to prevent serious tears.

7. Episiotomies can hurt for weeks and even months after delivery. This is not what the postpartum experience should be. One of the most wonderful things about the birthing

experience is the fleeting nature of the pain. After birth, though the mother may feel a little hungry or tired, there is little to attest to the fact that the body has just been through the ordeal of labor. The mother, following a normal and natural birth, feels whole and healthy; nature intends her to feel good because she now must devote her energies to a dependent baby. Episiotomies can take this feeling of energy and well-being away from women.

8. It has not been proved that full-term babies are injured by delivery without episiotomy. Their heads are quite able to withstand the pressure of the perineum.

9. Episiotomies can become infected, slowing down the mother's recovery process even further.

10. Proponents of the episiotomy seem to think that the birth outlet is somehow "flawed" and is in need of medical correction. I believe women's bodies were made perfectly to handle normal deliveries. I believe strongly in the wisdom "If it ain't broke don't fix it." Care providers should not interfere with nature unless there is a problem.

11. Women who have had episiotomies are more likely to suffer from painful intercourse after recovery from the birth.

12. The volume of blood loss with an episiotomy can be significant and is often greater than a tear, certainly greater than with an intact perineum.

HOW TO AVOID THIS PROCEDURE

The best way to avoid an episiotomy is by choosing a nurse-midwife (most midwives are trained in birth without episiotomy) or by using a doctor who does *not* do them routinely. As we mentioned earlier, if you're serious about avoiding one, do not choose a doctor who performs them on 98 percent of his patients. He or she is not going to skip *you*. You are much more likely to avoid an episiotomy by using a midwife who has been trained to safely avoid these cuts than by using a doctor who has been trained to believe women can't deliver without them.

If you aren't able to find a midwife, then talk to your doctor

about your feelings. Tell him or her you want to avoid an episiotomy. Ask if he or she will agree to cut only in an emergency,
such as a sudden drop in the baby's heart rate, necessitating
quick delivery, or if a tear is starting on your perineum. You
might also ask the doctor to try for a midline episiotomy if a cut
does turn out to be necessary. I would, however, caution you
against using a doctor who agrees to skip the episiotomy in your
case but who is not accustomed to delivering this way. You may
be more likely to tear because the doctor may not take any steps
to avoid it. For example, he or she may try to deliver you flat
on your back with legs in stirrups, a position that only increases
the chances of tearing.

No matter whom you choose to deliver your baby, there are
ways that you can prepare your body and increase your chances
of an intact perineum.

Squatting: Practice squatting every day. This stretches and
stimulates circulation to the pelvic area. This exercise will also
help you if you want to sit, squat, or kneel for the delivery (all
good positions to assume for an intact perineum).

Kegel Exercise: Exercising the pelvic floor muscles will make
them stronger and more supple. The Kegel exercise is named
after the doctor who originally prescribed it as an alternative to
surgery for nonpregnant women with urinary incontinence. The
best way to locate the pelvic floor muscles is by trying to stop
the flow of urine midstream when you are urinating. The muscle
power you use to do this is the same that you need to exercise
in preparation for childbirth. It's difficult to stop the flow of urine
if the bladder is very full or if you're very pregnant, so wait and
try it near the end of the flow. Then release, and continue to
urinate.

Now that you've got the hang of it, you can practice anywhere,
anytime. (In the beginning, you may get a strange look on your
face while trying to do them, so don't practice in front of anyone
whose friendship you value!) Think of your pelvic floor as an
elevator—contract the muscles and try to lift the elevator; then

hold for one minute. Then slowly release and let the elevator down to the ground floor slowly, not with a thud. You should do at least twenty to thirty a day for maximum benefit. I know this sounds like a lot, so try to break them up. Do a few every time you go to the bathroom. Here's a plus to keep in mind: the Kegel exercise won't make you sore and has an unexpected benefit— better sex. Some women experience orgasms for the first time, or more frequently, after they've toned their pelvic floor muscles with the Kegel exercise.

The reason the Kegel works so well for the avoidance of an episiotomy or tear is that it teaches you where the vaginal muscles are, how to tighten them, and how to relax them, allowing the baby to exit gently.

Perineal Massage: During the last few weeks of pregnancy, practice perineal massage to stretch the skin and tissues around the vagina. The perineum is the area between the vagina and rectum. This is the area that would be cut during an episiotomy. Perineal massage can help you to prepare for birth without a cut or tear. It duplicates some of the pressure and burning you will feel when the baby's head reaches the birth outlet and thus gives you a better idea of what birth will be like. This may help you to relax at the birth, a key to keeping your perineum intact. Try to massage the perineum once a day and within a week you'll feel the increased flexibility. If you have already had an episiotomy with a previous childbirth, you may have to pay extra attention to the scar tissue you have. It will not stretch as easily as the rest of your vagina and perineal area. You may massage the area alone or with the help of your partner. Having a partner is a lot easier but not always convenient or possible. Some couples may feel uncomfortable with the exercise, and the woman may prefer to do the massage alone. Here are some hints, no matter which way you approach the massage.

Alone: Take a warm bath to relax. Wash your hands. Find a private place to sit and use a mirror to find the vagina and perineum and see what they look like. With vitamin E oil, vegetable oil, KY jelly, or cocoa butter on your fingers and perineum, place your thumbs about one inch into your vagina. Press downward and out to the sides, gently stretching the vaginal area with each downward motion. Keep stretching until you feel a burning sensation. Give in to the feeling of pressure; try not to tighten up in response to it, but think instead about opening up. The feeling during the pushing stage will be similar but intensified. Keep applying pressure for a minute or so. Slowly and gently massage the lower half of the vagina, rubbing back and forth. As you continue the massage, try to pull gently outward on the lowest part of the vagina. This is where the baby's head will push through during birth.

With a partner: Read the section above. Have your partner wash his hands. He then applies oil to your perineum and his fingers. Your partner should use one or two fingers (index or thumb) to massage and stretch, as explained above. Tell your partner when you begin to feel the burn. He should hold that amount of pressure for two minutes, then massage the lower half of the vagina, gently pulling outward as he sweeps back and forth from side to side.

Warm Compresses: At the delivery, ask the nurse to give you sterile four-by-four gauze pads to use on the perineum. Use warm tap water or sterile saline solution to wet them and have them placed on the perineum as soon as the baby's head starts to show. It feels wonderful and helps relax the perineum. If you are using a midwife, she will probably apply warm compresses without your having to ask.

Delivery Position: Avoid stirrups. Putting a woman's legs up in stirrups stretches the perineum and makes it that much more difficult to get the baby out without a tear. In the recent study cited earlier, of episiotomies at the University of California, San Francisco, the rate of episiotomies was twice as high for delivery room births as for labor room births. Using a delivery table, there were 284 cases of rectal injury reported, as opposed to only 67 cases in a labor bed. (In almost all the cases, the rectal injury occurred in conjunction with an episiotomy.) Even if your doctor insists on a delivery room, ask if the stirrups can be left off. Agree to use them for any possible suturing afterward if this helps your case.

Try to deliver upright at a forty-five-degree angle when you're pushing (it's easier to push downhill than uphill). Standing, squatting or supported squatting, kneeling, and on hands and knees are also less likely to cause tears because it is in these positions that the birth canal is open widest and the pressure is most even. The pelvic area, including the perineum, is relaxed, and pushing with gravity is easier.

Relaxed Breathing: As the baby's head begins to show, hard pushing combined with breath holding to the rhythm of the cheerleading shouts of the doctors and nurses around you can be exhausting and even frustrating. It's better to push when you feel the urge and to concentrate on the messages from your body. Open your mouth and relax your jaw as you push; this will help to relax your vagina. If you feel a burning or tearing sensation, slow down by relaxing your breathing, panting if necessary. Push gently if you feel painful burning. Don't concentrate on pushing. The uterus will do this by itself. Think about opening up and releasing the pelvic floor muscles. There should be no rigid time limit set on this stage of pushing as long as the baby's heartbeat remains normal.

Encouragement: The caregiver should encourage you and support your efforts. If possible, reach down and feel the head of the baby as it crowns. This should reassure you that you are still intact and not splitting apart, and that the baby is on his or her way out at long last.

Delivery of the Head: The head should be delivered slowly. When the baby's head starts to crown, the midwife will place one hand lightly on it to make sure it doesn't slide out too quickly and then help to ease it out as slowly as possible. The delivering mother should deliver at a pace that makes her feel she won't tear. Slow down if it doesn't feel right to you. As long as the baby's heartbeat is fine, you can deliver the head as slowly as you like. Let the head crown through three, four, or five contractions. It's not easy, but it's worth if it you can avoid a tear or episiotomy.

Perineal Massage During the Delivery: The midwife might do perineal massage during the second stage, to continue to stretch with her own fingers a little more than the baby has stretched. Also, putting pressure on the floor of the vagina helps some women to get a better sense of where to push the baby during this stage of labor.

IVs

Intravenous infusions of sterile water with sugar, salt, and other minerals are routine for laboring women in most hospitals. A plastic catheter is put into a vein and taped in place. The IV is often used as a precautionary measure so that the woman won't become dehydrated or exhausted during labor. The reason a woman might become dehydrated or weak is due to another hospital policy that forbids her food and drink during labor and delivery. (See the section on food restriction during labor on pages 172–174.)

WHEN YOU MAY NEED THIS PROCEDURE

The IV can be a great help and sometimes lifesaving if surgical intervention is anticipated; if the woman is likely to bleed heavily after delivery (this might happen in the case of an oxytocin-induced labor, twins, or prolonged labor); or if a woman is dehydrated from vomiting, diarrhea, a long labor, or having food withheld due to medical regulations. Once the IV is in place, it is easy to get drugs quickly to the patient. IVs certainly have their place when women are at high risk for emergencies (high blood pressure, maternal disease) or if certain risk factors develop during labor such as fetal distress.

WHY YOU MIGHT NOT WANT THIS PROCEDURE

IVs are cumbersome and inconvenient. Psychologically, they can make you feel as though you're sick (not an encouraging thought for a woman who is about to face twelve hours of hard work). Nobody likes to be stuck with a needle or connected to a bag of fluids for twelve to fourteen hours. It's uncomfortable and restricts movement. If combined with a monitor, it can make you feel "wired for sound." The IV conveys the message that labor is an illness and that lots of intervention will be necessary in order to survive. Again, that's not a very positive message. A woman's labor is something like a marathon for runners. No one would consider hooking runners up to an IV to give them extra energy during their run. Furthermore, an IV can always be started if the situation changes from normal to problematic.

HOW TO AVOID THIS PROCEDURE

1. If you eat lightly and drink fruit juices during the early stages of labor, you probably won't need an IV for sustenance and strength. Unfortunately, some hospitals do not allow the woman to eat or drink during any stage of labor. See the section on food restriction during labor below.
2. If your doctor insists on the IV because he or she wants it in place in case of emergency, then ask about a Heparin Lock. The Heparin Lock is a plastic needle inserted into a vein and taped in place. It is not attached to an IV line or pole. The vein is hooked up and available if needed in a crisis, but you have the freedom to move around unhampered until that time.
3. Make sure to discuss IV concerns *before* you go into labor. This is one of those issues you will want to clear up during your pregnancy.

Food Restriction During Labor

Most hospitals insist that laboring mothers neither eat nor drink. They often allow only ice chips. Even if no high-risk indications are suspected, anesthesiologists don't want women eating or drinking during labor just in case they have to perform an emergency C-section under general anesthesia (when a full stomach can cause vomiting and possible aspiration into the lungs). Realistically, many women start labor following a full meal, so the restrictions of the hospital are hard to enforce. Furthermore, accident patients are often brought into the hospital for emergencies, and *they've* eaten. I think that it makes about as much sense to advise people not to eat if they're going to drive a car that day as it does to advise pregnant women not to eat if they're going into labor that day. The chances of needing emergency surgery under general anesthesia are probably about equal. Furthermore, according to a 1987 article in *Childbirth Educator*, written by the president of the American Foundation for Maternal and Child Health, there is no documented case of aspiration in a properly anesthetized delivering woman (full stomach or not).

WHEN YOU MAY NEED THIS PROCEDURE

Food restriction may be justified in high-risk pregnancies that could end with general anesthesia in an emergency cesarean. This would ostensibly lower the risks for anesthesia complications. If a woman is vomiting in labor, then restricting food and drink is sometimes the only way to stop the vomiting. At this point, an IV is essential.

WHY YOU MIGHT NOT WANT THIS PROCEDURE

The lack of food can weaken a woman just when she needs her strength. After the early stages of labor, most women would rather not eat anyway. But in the beginning, a little sustenance is a good idea. Light foods by mouth (crackers, tea with honey, hard candy) are easy to digest and give a woman energy. Soft drinks and fruit juices can help a woman get through her labor without needing an IV.

HOW TO AVOID THIS PROCEDURE

It can be really tough to avoid a procedure like this one if it is hospital policy. If possible, choose a practitioner who does not advocate it or a setting where food restriction is not practiced. It's always better to choose a practitioner and hospital or birth center that manages labor the way you like rather than constantly having to fight the system. If your practitioner or setting does not allow food, however, at least ask about hard candies or ice cubes made with fruit juice or raspberry-leaf tea. Perhaps these small energy boosters may be allowed.

Painkillers

Narcotics are often used in labor to help relax the mother and to "take the edge off the pain." In my experience, a good physician, nurse, midwife, or childbirth teacher giving hands-on care is worth more than any narcotic. A prepared, practiced, and relaxed woman is unlikely to feel she *needs* drugs. The most frequently used painkilling drug in obstetrics today is Demerol. It can be given intravenously or in the muscle.

WHEN YOU MAY NEED THIS PROCEDURE

Even women who prefer to labor without drugs may find that they have a change of heart during labor. If you do *need* a painkiller, you should obviously take it and not feel like a failure. For example, a woman with back labor or who is in severe pain may benefit from a painkiller. In back labor, all the pain is felt in the small of the back instead of in the lower abdomen. This pain tends to linger between contractions and so these women don't get a break between contractions as they would during normal labor contractions. Back labor is more common when the baby is presenting in the occiput posterior position (with his or her back against the mother's back). A woman who despite attempts on the part of the practitioner seems unable to cope with any of her contractions and unable to relax may also be a good candidate. Unfortunately, many women today are led to believe from the outset that labor will be too painful to handle on their own. This is a cultural bias and not a medical fact.

WHY YOU MIGHT NOT WANT THIS PROCEDURE

While Demerol helps to relax some women, it makes others feel too groggy to deal effectively with their contractions, and some women lose control of their labors as a result. Demerol can slow maternal respiration and circulation, suggesting that the fetus might also receive less oxygen and blood. Demerol crosses the placenta to the baby and can depress the baby's respiration at birth. In a study done at the University of Mississippi, one out of every four babies born to mothers who had been given this drug less than four hours before delivery needed resuscitation at birth (as reported by Doris Haire in "Drugs in Labor and Birth," *Childbirth Educator*, Spring 1987). Maternal side effects of Demerol are uncommon but can include sweating, dizziness, headache, nausea, and disorientation, among others.

In all there are about fourteen drugs that have been specifically approved for use in labor or delivery. This does not mean, however, that these drugs are guaranteed safe. A doctor is also free to prescribe to pregnant women drugs that have not been specifically okayed for that purpose. Ask about the drugs you are being offered or given. You have a right to know whether the drug has been approved for use in labor and delivery. You also have a right to know of all side effects and possible dangers associated with use of the drug.

HOW TO AVOID THIS PROCEDURE

Read Chapters 6 and 7 on labor and delivery, especially the tips on how to cope with painful contractions in the section on active labor, pages 138–140. Practice your relaxation and breathing exercises from childbirth class. Remember that the pain you feel is a positive force, bringing your baby closer to you. Let your practitioner know that you would like to avoid painkillers. Midwives look upon the pain of labor as a positive force and rarely use painkillers. Because the midwife's patients tend to feel secure, relaxed, and cared for, they usually don't need them. If you choose a doctor, try to locate one who does not use painkillers on the vast majority of patients.

Epidurals

Regional anesthetics include bupivacaine (Marcaine, Sensorcaine) and lidocaine (Xylocaine), among a number of others. They are given in the form of an epidural, spinal, saddle, or pudendal block or as a local shot for an episiotomy. Epidurals and spinal blocks numb women from the waist down. Saddle and pudendal blocks numb the perineal area. Why do so many women today end up with drugs and epidurals during labor and pregnancy? Pregnant women are sometimes told that their pain can decrease the oxygen supply to their babies. No research has ever confirmed this statement. Many women are also led to believe that the pain of childbirth will be so awful they won't be able to handle it on their own. This is untrue.

Recently, I spoke with an obstetrical anesthesiologist about epidurals and the improvements that had been made, which were impressive. Then I asked him how many women actually got through labor in his hospital without any anesthesia and found it was only about 15 percent. Most were multips (having a second or third baby). In our birth center, on the other hand, all mothers (except for the 12 percent who transfer to a hospital for complications), both first-timers and multips, manage to labor and deliver *without* painkillers or anesthesia. I asked why he thought so many women in his hospital needed anesthesia. He said that the patients got very little support from the nurses and doctors to labor without anesthesia. (This, again, shows how important attitudes and practices are.) When I am with a woman in labor, I try to help her through these difficult moments—not because I think women should "tough it out," but because I know that with a little encouragement and support they usually find the pain bearable and can use it as a positive force in the birth of their baby—and, perhaps most important, because birth without unnecessary drugs is *safer* for both mother and baby. Women in labor are very vulnerable to suggestion and need an experienced, confident person to *stay with them* to encourage and coach them. The word *midwife*, in fact, means "with the woman."

It is wrong to condemn the epidural across the board because, when necessary, it is by far the best form of anesthesia available for childbirth. If it is needed, it is always the anesthesia of choice. The point is that it is usually not needed. It is a cultural belief that women need epidurals to deliver, not a medical fact.

WHEN YOU MAY NEED THIS PROCEDURE

1. Severe back labor or complications may cause the woman a great deal of pain. With an epidural, the woman is awake and aware but without pain from navel to knees. Epidurals can be used from the middle of labor (about five centimeters through delivery).
2. The epidural can calm the woman who feels out of control due to the pain of labor. The drug can be allowed to wear off toward the end of labor so that the woman can push more effectively.
3. The epidural's effects can be stepped up so a C-section can be done or forceps used. (Medication is added via catheter so there is no further discomfort.)
4. The woman usually has no urge to push and therefore can more easily wait for those caring for her to arrive. On a busy labor floor, this makes for less rushing around and the staff can control the pace of everyone's births better.
5. The woman feels nothing and can be pleasant to everyone, including her coach, as labor progresses. She can even nap or sleep during the most difficult parts of labor, and yet she will be awake to receive her baby after birth.

6. If the woman is exhausted and very tense, epidurals will allow much more complete relaxation to occur, often helping the cervix to dilate.

7. If Pitocin is used to stimulate the labor and the woman can't cope with the intensity of the contractions that Pitocin causes, the epidural will give good pain relief.

WHY YOU MIGHT NOT WANT THIS PROCEDURE

On the down side, the epidural has many serious disadvantages:

1. An epidural often leads to longer labors.

2. Labors tend to slow down once an epidural is working, which may necessitate augmenting the labor with synthetic hormones. Pitocin is often used to speed up labor in these cases. (See the section on Pitocin, pages 180–181.)

3. Pitocin, a synthetic hormone, can, in turn, cause fetal distress and make other interventions more likely.

4. There is more postpartum urinary catheterization following epidurals, due to bladder dysfunction caused by the drug and/or the use of forceps.

5. There is a higher incidence of episiotomy.

6. Being numb, the mother is unable to bear down effectively during the pushing stage.

7. There is a higher incidence of tears and damage to the perineum (the mother cannot feel the usual burning sensation that lets her know how to control her pushing).

8. Forceps are used more frequently following an epidural because the woman can't push as effectively. (Furthermore, there is an increased risk of postdelivery hemorrhage after Pitocin and forceps have been used.)

9. There is an increased incidence of C-section after epidurals. (Pelvic muscles may become limp. An epidural can lead to dysfunction of the pelvic muscles, which normally rotate the baby into the proper position for delivery.)

10. Though it rarely occurs, the needle may puncture the dura,

causing spinal fluid to leak and resulting in severe headache with nausea, vomiting, and vertigo. Treatment involves lying flat on the back in bed, as sitting up makes the symptoms worse. Obviously, a woman in this condition will have a very difficult time breast-feeding or enjoying her newborn.

11. Extremely rare but serious complications have been reported, ranging from convulsions to loss of sensation or paralysis of the lower limbs. A more common serious complication is maternal hypotension, which is a drop in maternal blood pressure. The blood-pressure drop may mean that the fetus is no longer getting enough oxygen. In the mother, it can cause nausea and fainting.

12. The safest way for a healthy woman to give birth is without anesthesia. Period. It is safer for her and safer for her baby. Epidurals are wonderful for complications, but they are not the best thing for normal deliveries.

HOW TO AVOID THIS PROCEDURE

1. Know as much as you can about the drugs that may be offered to you. Ask your doctor or midwife for information on side effects and dangers. Find out whether the drug is approved for use in pregnancy, labor, or lactation.

2. Choose a caregiver who doesn't always rely on drugs as a labor-management technique. Midwives are much less likely to suggest an epidural than obstetricians are.

3. Depend on your coach and, we hope, your caregiver for the support you need to make it through labor without a drug.

4. Remind yourself that drugs are there if necessary, but since they have risks, they should be used as a last resort.

5. Think of the pain you feel as a positive force that helps your baby to be born.

6. Think of the thousands of other women all over the world who are laboring with you.

7. Relax between contractions so you can face the next wave calmly.

Pitocin

Pitocin is a powerful synthetic hormone that induces contractions. Pitocin is used to begin labor or to move a slow labor along more quickly. It is an FDA-approved drug for labor and delivery.

WHEN YOU MAY NEED THIS PROCEDURE

- When labor is weak or unproductive
- When the membranes have been ruptured for a long time but no labor has begun
- When the baby is weeks overdue and no labor has begun
- In the case of placental dysfunction, when the placenta ceases to nourish the baby and delivery would be safer than staying in the womb
- If the mother has high blood pressure that is getting worse
- To prevent hemorrhaging after birth when the uterus is not contracting well enough on its own

WHY YOU MIGHT NOT WANT THIS PROCEDURE

Pitocin can cause the contractions to come too close together. They can be, unlike normal contractions, excessively long and strong. During a contraction—whether normal or synthetically induced—oxygen-carrying blood vessels constrict. After the contraction, oxygen supplies are replenished and the fetus can therefore receive a fairly constant flow of oxygen both during and in between contractions. Without much space between hard contractions, however, there is little time for the fetus's oxygen supply to be replenished. Pitocin has also been associated occasionally with damage to the uterus if the contractions are too intense. According to Doris Haire's article in *Childbirth Educator* cited earlier, British research has indicated that births induced with Pitocin lead to a higher percentage of jaundiced babies. This theory has not been tested in the United States.

I know of *no* contraindication to the use of Pitocin to stop postpartum hemorrhage. It saves lives and should be used to prevent excess blood loss.

HOW TO AVOID THIS PROCEDURE

1. Walk, stand, or sit throughout most of your labor. This should help you to progress in labor unassisted.
2. Make sure you agree with your doctor that induction of labor is necessary. If you are being induced because you're late, double-check your dates with the doctor's. If there is some disagreement about your dates, perhaps you can suggest an ultrasound examination to check on the baby's size and gestational age before agreeing to induction.
3. Ask about more natural methods of labor induction: a long walk, an enema, intercourse. Similarly, once in labor, you can try some nondrug methods of speeding things up: walking around, nipple stimulation, an enema.
4. See pages 142–144 for more information on induction of labor.

Continuous Electronic Fetal Monitoring

The baby's heartbeat and the mother's contractions can be continuously monitored by machine throughout labor and recorded on a printout. The monitoring can give the doctor or midwife good information on how well the baby is tolerating the stress of labor. A change in the baby's heart-rate patterns, especially as they relate to contractions, can indicate that the baby is having some trouble.

WHEN YOU MAY NEED THIS PROCEDURE

For Pitocin-induced labors or for high-risk babies, such as prematures, babies of diabetic mothers or of drug-addicted mothers, and unusually small babies, the monitor's information can be lifesaving. It can help the doctor decide on an emergency C-section when necessary. On a busy day, with the help of a monitor, a nurse can keep track of several laboring mothers at the same time. The coach can look at the monitor screen and predict when contractions are beginning, peaking, and ending; he can use this information to help his partner cope better with her contractions. In today's litigious society, there is one other practical reason for the use of a monitor: the printout can be used as evidence to support either the OB's or the parents' case.

WHY YOU MIGHT NOT WANT THIS PROCEDURE

A fetal monitor confines the mother to bed and makes her feel as though she's sick. This can slow down the progress of labor, since the mother is not able to walk around and may feel uncomfortable lying in bed strapped to a machine. The slowdown of her labor can lead, of course, to other interventions, including an internal monitor, rupture of the membranes, IV, Pitocin, and more.

The coach and doctors and nurses sometimes appear more interested in watching the monitor than in helping the mother. Little attention may be paid to the mother's feelings or complaints. Even though we know the monitor is not very accurate at predicting the strength of a contraction, caregivers often rely more heavily on the monitor than on the mother's own description of how it feels. I sometimes think that the mother could be under the bed instead of in it and no one would notice as long as the printout remained good!

Ideally, use of the monitor should lower the rate of medical intervention in labor and delivery. Unfortunately, since the monitor has been in such heavy use, medical intervention, specifically the C-section, has been very much on the *increase*. Furthermore, continuous electronic fetal monitoring has never been proved to be beneficial to low-risk women and babies. As a matter of fact, two studies show that nurses listening with fetascopes intermittently were able to identify problems as well as monitors were. The group monitored by these nurses also had less Pitocin and fewer C-sections or forceps deliveries than the group monitored by machine. The difference may be due to the very basic need we all have to be cared for and touched by a person rather than a machine.

HOW TO AVOID THIS INTERVENTION

1. Ask that the monitor be used on arrival and then removed so you can continue to labor with freedom of movement. If necessary, you can be hooked up again for another check on the baby later.
2. Talk to your doctor or midwife about using the monitor only if you fall into a high-risk category, are having a difficult labor, or are receiving Pitocin.
3. Every fifteen or twenty minutes, have the baby's heartbeat checked during a contraction with a hand-held Doppler to pick up any problems. Just because you don't want continuous electronic fetal monitoring doesn't mean you don't want *anything*. There *is* a safe, intermediate step.

Forceps

Tonglike instruments called forceps are used occasionally to pull the baby down through the birth canal while the mother is pushing.

WHEN YOU MAY NEED THIS PROCEDURE

- During a prolonged second stage (pushing) that has begun to cause fetal distress
- When an epidural or other anesthesia has made pushing ineffective
- At a premature delivery

WHY YOU MIGHT NOT WANT THIS PROCEDURE

Use of forceps necessitates a large episiotomy. Even with a cut, further tearing of the vagina and cervix can occur. The metal clamps can squeeze the baby's head, causing bruises and small indentations. (These will disappear in a few days.) Unskilled or incorrect use of forceps, however, may result in skull fracture, eye injury, facial paralysis, and even brain damage. Tissue damage to the mother's bladder or urethra is also possible.

HOW TO AVOID THIS PROCEDURE

See Chapter 7, page 152, for tips on how to deal effectively with the second stage of labor. With proper preparation and a willingness to try various positions, you should be able to push the baby out without use of forceps. You will also want to avoid an epidural or other regional pain block, which can decrease your pushing effectiveness. Talk with your doctor or midwife prior to delivery about any time limits that may be imposed on the second stage. Try to choose a practitioner who allows you to push as long as fetal heart tones are good and progress is being made, rather than one who resorts to forceps after your one hour of pushing time is up.

Cesarean Births

More than one-fourth of all births in the United States today are by cesarean. The medical community and consumers are still struggling to determine why this is so and how we can change. Certainly, the high cesarean rate is due in part to today's litigious environment, where suing and being sued have become a way of life. The threat of malpractice suits plays a role in the thinking of every obstetrician and midwife. You need to know this in order to understand what makes midwives and doctors tick. As we said before, 70 percent of obstetricians have been sued. The most common reason for an obstetrician to be sued is *failure to do a timely cesarean.*

The premiums for obstetricians for malpractice insurance are between $40,000 and $200,000 a year, depending upon location and number of deliveries performed each year. (Midwives pay far, far lower rates, around $5,000 a year, because only 6 percent of midwives have been sued.) So one can easily imagine how an obstetrician might feel if a certain point in labor or pregnancy arises when there *could be* a risk to the baby. Even if the risk seems very small, a recent lawsuit or knowledge of a friend being sued in similar circumstances is likely to cause the practitioner to react conservatively.

There are always risks and benefits that must be weighed during pregnancy and birth. Decisions must be made all along the way, and it is not always clear or certain what *will happen*. Mother Nature is trickier than that. Practitioners can project only what is *most likely to happen*, based on past experiences, statistical studies, and even gut feelings. This can provide very anxious moments for the physician or midwife.

WHEN YOU MAY NEED THIS PROCEDURE

There is, of course, a place for the C-section, which can be a lifesaving procedure for mothers and babies. I should know— I've had all four of my children by cesarean. I'm a small woman, only about five feet tall, while my husband stands six feet two. Together we produce *large* babies (my last one, Annie, weighed 9 lbs. 8 oz.) who need to come out of my very small pelvis. When I had my first child twenty-one years ago, the C-section rate was only 7 percent and my surgery was disappointingly necessary. At that time the rule was: once a cesarean, always a cesarean, so my subsequent children were all delivered the same way. Fortunately, this rule is no longer observed as strictly as it once was.

Parents have to trust their caretakers to assess the baby's well-being at the time of delivery and make that decision about surgical birth. Reasons for a C-section include *cephalo-pelvic disproportion* (CPD), meaning a baby too large for the mother's pelvis; *transverse lie* (the baby is lying horizontally) or *breech presentation* (the baby is bottom- or feet-first); *failure to progress in labor*; *fetal distress*; *prolapsed cord*, meaning that the umbilical cord has dropped down ahead of the baby and is cutting off the baby's oxygen supply (this demands immediate intervention); *placenta previa*, a condition in which the placenta covers the cervix (when the cervix opens, part of the placenta over the cervix begins to bleed heavily); *abruptio placenta* (the placenta separates from the uterus and decreases fetal oxygen supply and causes hemorrhage); *genital herpes* (the baby could become infected during a vaginal birth); *maternal disease* such as toxemia, diabetes, high blood pressure, or heart disease (may make labor and vaginal delivery too stressful for mother and baby).

If you have been under the care of a nurse-midwife, and she decides during the labor that you may need a cesarean, the consulting physician will be contacted. He or she will begin to assess and manage the labor and delivery. The CNM and MD, who are accustomed to working together as a team, make this transition from one caregiver to another as smooth as possible, so that the woman feels that a continuity of care is being provided. The MD/CNM team is sensitive to the needs of the mother and works together to support the woman whose plans for delivery have changed dramatically. Your midwife may remain by your side during this operation. Exactly what role she plays will depend on her practice and the hospital in question. She may take on the role of an assisting physician or a nursing role, or she may assume a coaching role (emotional support only), or she may not be at the delivery at all. Ask in advance what she will be able to do in the event of a cesarean.

Usually, unless fetal distress is sudden and severe, the mother can be awake for a C-section. The mother is given an epidural for the surgery, which numbs her from the navel down, but she is still very much alert. Occasionally, an epidural isn't possible, due to time constraints, and she must be given general anesthesia. (It takes about one-half hour to administer an epidural and wait for it to take effect.)

In either case, C-section is not the delivery most women plan for, and for some women it is one of their biggest fears. It is very scary to face this operation—mothers fear for both their own safety and the safety of their babies. The operating room is foreign territory and rules of behavior change dramatically. Suddenly, the friendly faces disappear and serious, masked faces take their place. The nurses and doctors doing the surgery wear sterile gowns and caps, gloves and shoe covers. You'll see lots of monitors, IVs, oxygen masks. You'll be hooked up to machines to monitor your blood pressure, oxygen level, and heart rate. You look and feel wired. The feeling of being totally dependent on the health-care team around you is disconcerting. The mother and coach can look to the anesthesiologist for support and direction at this time. He or she can explain what is happening and how it is going to feel step by step. The anesthesiologist can provide wonderful support and confidence to the parents at this very stressful time.

What can the coach do during a section? Make good eye contact with the mother and ask the anesthesiologist where you can touch the mother: face, shoulder, arm, hand. Keep this physical contact. It gives the mother a feeling of being connected to someone who loves her. That support is invaluable.

Getting the baby delivered by cesarean section takes about ten to twenty minutes. In another twenty to thirty minutes, the surgeon will have closed the incision. At the delivery you can't see the birth because a screen is placed across your midsection. The baby is first given to the neonatologist or pediatrician and nurses to evaluate on a separate table. This unit will have an overhead heater, warm blankets, oxygen, and suction—everything needed to resuscitate a depressed newborn. If the baby is normal and healthy, he or she can be treated like any other newborn and will usually be brought to the parents to hold. The baby that needs special help will be transferred immediately to the intermediate- or intensive-care nursery for care and testing. Most hospitals will allow the father to accompany the baby there if he wishes.

After delivery, the mother will be transferred to the recovery room until the epidural anesthesia wears off. During this time, if the baby's condition is normal, it is often a good time to try nursing or holding the baby. While you are still under the influence of the epidural, there will be little postoperative pain. If the baby is kept in the nursery (due to routine or to get special help), a Polaroid picture can be taken to the mother. Usually the father can go to the nursery and bring periodic reports back to the mother.

It takes a certain strength to go through a cesarean and a good deal of courage. There is a special place in my heart for all those mothers who need to give birth this way. It is a sacrifice that you make for your baby's sake, and that is the beginning of motherhood.

WHY YOU MIGHT NOT WANT THIS PROCEDURE

It seems pretty obvious that no one would *want* a surgical birth if it weren't necessary. Here, though, are some of the specific disadvantages of C-sections.

1. All surgery carries with it certain inherent risks, from infection to death.
2. The mother may have to lie flat to avoid headaches after a spinal anesthetic.
3. The recovery period is much slower for the mother and can inhibit breast-feeding and early bonding.
4. The C-section may depress the mother. She may feel cheated out of a normal delivery, or like a failure because she delivered surgically.
5. A cesarean is much more expensive than a vaginal birth and requires more time in the hospital for recovery, another expense.
6. Vaginal birth is better for the mother because there is a lower risk of infection, less postpartum bleeding, and no anesthesia complications.
7. Vaginal birth is better for the baby because the pressure on the baby of being squeezed through the birth canal causes some of the fetal lung fluid to be expressed from the upper airways, making it easier for the baby to begin breathing spontaneously right after birth.
8. A planned cesarean performed before the mother actually goes into labor can result in premature birth.

HOW TO AVOID THIS PROCEDURE

1. A midwife is less likely to call for a cesarean. Of course, she cannot avoid one in the case of serious problems, but she is less likely to rush into one for the more subjective reason of prolonged labor or based on the subjective decision that the baby is too large for the mother's pelvis.
2. Whether you use a midwife or a doctor, try to find out how many of the practitioner's patients end up with cesareans. This usually indicates the speed with which this caregiver resorts to surgical methods for birth.
3. Don't go to the hospital too early in labor. The longer you are there, the more likely someone will decide you've been in labor too long.
4. If a C-section is suggested for a nonemergency reason, be sure to ask for the medical reasons behind the decision, plus what will happen if you wait a little longer. If you are not emotionally able to hold a rational discussion like this during labor, your coach should be the one to ask questions, so that you and he can at least understand the situation you are now in.
5. Consider your birthing options and talk about cesareans with your doctor or midwife during prenatal visits. This way, you'll be prepared to face everything that may come up during the labor and delivery.
6. Take a childbirth education course with your coach or other support person. Educate yourself so you can prepare for the best delivery available.
7. Take good care of yourself during pregnancy. Get excellent prenatal care, eat well, and stay fit with a regular exercise program.
8. If you have negative feelings, extreme fears, and/or a terrible prior birth experience, talk with your midwife or doctor to work through these feelings so that you can be ready for your labor and birth.

9

You and Your Baby
at Birth

The first few days with a newborn are both a happy and an anxious time for new parents. On the one hand, parents are deliriously happy with their new little one. On the other hand, they are often consumed with worry about everything from the baby's cold hands to the shape of his head to the first diaper change. This chapter should alleviate some of those early worries and help you ease into your new role as a parent.

Bonding Made Simple

Most babies are very alert for the first hour or two after birth, if the mothers haven't had drugs during labor. Unless there is a problem with the baby at birth, newborns belong with their parents. Babies respond to their mothers' voices. Babies who are touched, rocked, and cuddled thrive and grow better than those left in their bassinets. At birth, they need to be dried, warmed, and stimulated with lots of skin-to-skin contact. A baby placed on the mother's chest will get the human contact he seeks and the mother, likewise, will be reassured by the feel of this lively and healthy baby. Mothers instinctively talk to and rub their babies, rocking them to provide comfort. This is just what a baby needs at birth.

Unfortunately, this kind of mother-infant contact has not always been allowed to take place. Recently, hospitals and caretakers have become much more aware of the positive benefits of allowing mother and child to bond, so it is now more common to have the mother hold her baby soon after birth. The first time I saw a mother have unlimited access to her baby was at a home birth I attended soon after my graduation from midwifery school. The mother was giving birth for the first time, but the minute the baby was halfway out and crying, she instinctively reached down and picked the baby up from my hands. The rest of his body slid out and she lifted the child to her chest and began rocking, cuddling, and talking to the crying baby. This mother was doing something that came naturally to her, and it was working beautifully. This is the way birth has gone on for centuries, since the beginning of time. We can all learn from this pattern of noninterference and observation. In fact, the more we learn about newborns at birth, the more this natural pattern makes sense.

A newborn will open his eyes and look at the mother, especially in response to her voice. When a mother holds a baby in her arms the distance between them is about twelve inches, which is just perfect because that's how far away the baby can see. The baby should have a chance to make eye contact with the mother, and bright lights should be kept away from the baby, whose eyes are adjusting. It helps a mother fall in love with her baby when the baby turns and looks at her. It makes sense to enhance that process whenever possible. Leaving the baby with the mother also helps to keep the child warm. The mother's body is like a natural radiator.

The cord can be left intact until it stops pulsating. When pulsation stops, then it can be clamped and cut. There is no need to cut the cord immediately. Letting it pulse gives the baby a little extra blood and is in keeping with the belief in no interference without reason. If the baby is born with the cord tightly wrapped around his neck, however, the cord will be cut right away. If it's loosely wrapped, as it very frequently is, it can be slipped over the baby's head. If the baby's respiration is depressed at birth, she can be resuscitated first and then the cord can be clamped. In a hospital, however, the baby must be moved to a table for resuscitation efforts (there's no room on the delivery table) and so the cord must be clamped before resuscitation efforts can begin. All babies should be continually observed during that first hour after birth. This can be done anywhere a normal birth takes place—at home, the birth center, or the hospital. For normal babies, this observation can be done with the baby in the mother's arms.

I like to leave the baby on the mother's chest until the placenta is delivered and while the mother is being sutured if that's necessary. If the baby needs a little oxygen or suctioning, this can be done on the bed. Some babies need this extra help to breathe, especially if the baby has extra fluid in the nose and throat. Only when the baby is taken away with no explanation do parents get upset. And I don't blame them. Good newborn care includes communication with the parents, always.

Obviously, some of the best-laid plans for a gentle, family-centered birth can change radically if there is a problem with the baby at birth. The most common problem would be breathing difficulties, which can range from mild to severe. You may barely be able to touch your baby at birth if there is a serious problem; the baby may be whisked off to a nursery for medical care until the problem is resolved. Many mothers in this situation worry—among other things—about bonding. Bonding is a process that begins at birth and continues throughout life. You will bond and reconnect and love and attach to this child as he grows and changes all through your life. Early bonding at delivery simply makes the first step as easy as possible for babies and their parents. However, mothers bond with their babies under all kinds of circumstances: through the portholes of Isolettes, and via photos if the baby is transferred to another hospital facility. Early bonding is a small step in a continuum, and it should be encouraged. Even parents of the sickest of babies will want to be with that child and to be involved in the baby's care. Recognition of the needs of the parents is important and helps parents to turn their attention to the baby's problems and needs.

Apgar Scores

All newborns are "rated" at delivery, at one minute after birth, and again at five minutes after birth. There are five categories: color, heart rate, respiration, muscle tone, and reflex irritability. A score of 0, 1, or 2 is given in each category and then totaled. A score of 7 to 10 is considered good and indicates a healthy baby. The rating can be very subjective, however, because it does reflect the caregiver's management of the labor and birth. Apgar scores are more accurate when they are done by a nurse or pediatrician rather than by the midwife or obstetrician who performed the delivery.

Eye Drops and Other Hospital Procedures

Silver nitrate drops, or erythromycin or tetracycline ointments, are put in a newborn's eyes within the first hour after birth. This is done to prevent possible blindness, which can be the result of a baby born to a mother with gonorrhea. All babies in the United States receive this treatment because tests to detect gonorrhea are not accurate enough to pinpoint *all* women who have the disease. You may ask, however, that the drops not be given immediately after birth, so that your baby has a few minutes for a clear-eyed look at the world and his parents. (The medication can blur the baby's vision for a little while.) The antibiotic ointments are less irritating to the newborn's eyes than the silver nitrate drops. Talk with your practitioner about which medication will be used.

An injection of vitamin K is usually given to newborns to help their blood clot. Babies do not make vitamin K in their intestines until about five days after birth when there is enough normal intestinal bacteria. To help "cover" for this time, babies are usually given an injection soon after delivery. This is especially important if you are planning to have a boy circumcised.

The baby will also be weighed and measured, and his footprint will be taken for hospital identification.

How Babies Look

Newborns have a very distinctive look. Right at birth, they may have a bluish color that quickly changes to pink as they cry. The head may be especially blue if it took a few minutes for the shoulders to be born into the world. If the baby was born with the cord around her neck (as are 30 percent of babies), her oxygen supply may have been pinched off momentarily and her face can remain blue a few minutes longer, even though she's breathing normally. As long as she's vigorous, the pink color should return to the face within a few minutes.

The hands and feet of a newborn will stay bluish for a while after delivery. For now, the baby's blood supply is being pulled toward the vital organs—brain, heart, and lungs. This is normal.

The baby at birth will be wet from the amniotic fluid and slippery with vernix caseosa, the greasy substance produced by the baby to protect his skin from the last nine months underwater. The newborn may also have some of the mother's blood on him, from a tear or episiotomy. The baby will be dried off to keep him from losing heat to the relatively cold air (he has just switched from a ninety-nine-degree environment to a seventy-eight-degree room). There is no urgent need to bathe the newborn. The baby can simply be wiped off. He is not dirty.

Usually, the head is molded into an elongated shape, especially with the first delivery. The bones of a baby's skull are soft and not firmly joined together, which allows the head to fit the size of the mother's pelvis. Some babies therefore have fairly pointy heads, especially if they were in a posterior position at birth. Bald babies can also look startling because their lack of hair makes it much easier to see the overlapping lines where the skull bones connect.

Body hair is often present—on the baby's ears, low on the forehead, across the shoulders and arms. This is not permanent hair. It is called lanugo and will fall out in the first two months. At the opposite end of the spectrum, some babies are hairless and totally bald. This, too, will change.

Why Babies Cry at Birth

Babies respond to the lights, noise, cold air, and pressure change at the delivery by gasping for air and crying. This is the way they expand their lungs. The amount of force it takes to expand the lungs for the first time is greater than the amount of force needed to keep them open once inflated. A baby's first cry can provide the force needed to get those airways open and working.

Meconium

Soon after delivery (sometimes at delivery), the baby will have a first bowel movement. This waste, called meconium, is black and tarlike. If meconium is present before the baby is born, she will need some special suctioning at delivery to keep the meconium from being pulled into the lungs. It may be necessary to empty the baby's stomach as well as suction her to make sure no meconium was ingested or aspirated. Some hospitals then routinely take a baby born with meconium to the nursery for observation.

When the baby passes meconium *after* birth, there is nothing to fear. Though it looks strange to the untrained eye, all is normal. Cleanup can be a chore, however!

Jaundice

About 30 percent of newborns get a yellow tinge to their skin known as jaundice. (They are not born with jaundice.) This normal newborn jaundice peaks at day three of life and then gradually subsides. It is caused by excess red blood cells that the baby needs while in the uterus but not after delivery. Normally, these cells are broken down and excreted through the liver, but sometimes this process is complicated by a blood incompatibility with the mother or by infection. In these cases, the bilirubin level (a measure of jaundice) rises drastically and can *in extreme cases* cause brain damage.

To prevent newborn jaundice from occurring, breast-feed every two to three hours in the first few days of life. Your colostrum (the precursor of breast milk) will help eliminate meconium from the intestines. Meconium contains bilirubin. Nursing the baby every few hours will keep the baby well hydrated, which also aids in eliminating excess jaundice. Bottle-feeding does this also. Exposing the baby's skin to sunlight through a closed window or to an ordinary lamp's light will reduce the level of jaundice. Undress the baby down to the diaper and place him face-down (to keep the light from the eyes) in the sun or lamp light. The baby will not get sunburned through glass and can be left in the light for hours at a time. You need to make sure, however, that the baby doesn't get overheated or chilled while in the light.

If you stay in the hospital for two to three days, the nurses and physicians will observe your baby for jaundice. If you leave on the day of delivery or if you deliver at a birth center or at home, the pediatrician or nurse-midwife will watch for jaundice on visits to the baby during the first few days of life. In between these visits, you can check for jaundice yourself. Look at the baby in daylight near a window. If you press the baby's nose and see that where the skin blanches it looks slightly yellow, your baby may have jaundice. Check the chest, arms, abdomen, and legs as well. Also look at the whites of the baby's eyes and the gums. A yellow, a bright yellow, or an orange cast to the skin or eyes should be reported to your pediatrician. If the baby gets lethargic, sleepy, and hot, and won't nurse, this also may be a sign of jaundice and the baby should be seen by your pediatrician. A blood test or two will be ordered to check bilirubin levels. At the worst, your baby may have to be treated in the hospital nursery under special lights to reduce the bilirubin level and prevent severe jaundice from occurring.

Breast-milk jaundice is an unusual occurrence. Babies with this condition have a slightly elevated bilirubin level while being breast-fed. It is not harmful to the baby. This type of jaundice does not occur in the first two or three days of life; it usually occurs after the first week. Most breast-feeding experts will not have a mother give up breast-feeding due to breast-milk jaundice. Breast-feeding is not the cause of severe jaundice—another cause should be looked for. If you are told to stop breast-feeding because of jaundice, it's wise to get a second opinion from a pediatrician who supports breast-feeding and who will give you an explanation of what is happening.

Circumcision

In this country, it has until recently been traditional practice to circumcise all male babies. Circumcision entails the removal of the foreskin from the end of the penis. This practice was based on beliefs and traditions, not medical facts. There has been a rethinking of the necessity for routine circumcision and new guidelines have been issued. The American Academy of Pediatrics (the national organization of pediatricians) no longer endorses routine circumcision. Why not? Because circumcision has not been proved to protect against infection or cancer of the penis, or cancer of the cervix in the female sex partner. Uncircumcised men and boys have no problem with personal hygiene. Furthermore, circumcision hurts (it is not done under any anesthesia), and there is no evidence that it hurts a baby any less than it would a grown man (a newborn just has limited ways of complaining). As with any surgery, there is always the risk of infection or injury.

Some parents worry about not circumcising because they think their child will look or feel different. Many parents are now making the decision *not* to circumcise, so your child will certainly not be the only one in school who looks the way he does. Uncircumcised children of circumcised fathers do not seem upset about being "different" either. If necessary, you can always explain, "Male babies used to be routinely circumcised, but then the medical community decided it wasn't a good idea anymore so we didn't do it to you." You can use this same explanation if an older brother in the house is circumcised. The fact that a father or older brother looks different should not stop you from learning new facts and changing for a better plan.

Based on the latest medical opinion, the only reason to circumcise a boy is religious belief or if the parents believe that they would feel emotionally unable to deal with a boy who is uncircumcised. If, in your mind, not circumcising your son is going to get in the way of relating comfortably to him, then you should consider having him circumcised.

Breast-feeding: A Prejudiced View

Breast-feeding is the best way to nourish a baby. Bottle-feeding is good, but the breast is better and should be encouraged whenever possible. Why?

1. Human milk is perfectly suited to a newborn. It is easy to digest and contains antibodies to help the baby fight infection.
2. For the first few days, the mother produces colostrum (a precursor of milk), which is also of benefit to her baby. It contains twice as much protein as later breast milk and is full of antibodies to help protect the baby from disease. The colostrum also aids the baby in the passing of meconium.
3. The milk is inexpensive, always available, and, as La Leche League says, comes in attractive containers.

4. Breast-feeding is easy. At the six-week checkup, I find that 96 percent of the women who delivered at our center are offering their babies only the breast.
5. When the baby sucks at the breast, it causes the uterus to contract, which minimizes blood loss and also helps your uterus to return to its nonpregnant size, a process called involution which takes about six weeks.
6. When a mother breast-feeds, she feels she is giving something to her baby no one else can give. It makes it easier for the mother to bond with her baby. When the baby thrives on her breast milk, this enhances the mother's self-esteem and she is rewarded for mothering well.

Below are some tips to make that first feeding go smoothly.

First Feeding Tips

Worrying about breast-feeding and about whether you have enough milk causes anxiety. Anxiety interferes with successful breast-feeding. You really need only two pieces of advice to breast-feed successfully: (1) relax and (2) feed the baby when she's hungry. (Hungry babies cry, open their mouths, and move their heads from side to side looking for a nipple to suck. This is called rooting.) Water and formula supplements are rarely needed. Since you probably won't be satisfied with these two tips alone, I'll give some more instructions to make breast-feeding even simpler.

I advise that you begin breast-feeding as soon after delivery as possible. Make sure you have good back support and hold the baby in a comfortable position. (See page 201 for position ideas.) The baby doesn't know a nipple by sight so you'll want to help him by following his mouth with your nipple. Hold the nipple between your index finger and thumb, and put it into the baby's mouth. Be sure to get the nipple well back inside. It won't choke him; it will stimulate his sucking reflex. You don't want him to suck just on the end of the nipple or you'll get very sore. (For information on sore nipples, see Chapter 10.) Part of the areola should also be in your baby's mouth. Let your baby suck for about ten minutes. Do not sit and watch a clock or set an alarm. This is a natural event, not a scientific experiment. After ten minutes or so, release the suction by inserting a finger into the baby's mouth. Switch breasts and let the baby nurse for ten minutes or more on the other side.

Tips for the Reluctant Feeder

Some babies are slow feeders, fall asleep, or don't seem to get the hang of breast-feeding right away. Here are some ideas to make feedings go more smoothly:

- Massage the baby's back, abdomen, and legs to stimulate the baby's rooting reflex.
- Be patient. The first few nursings can be awkward. You may feel that you need four hands—one to hold the nipple, one to hold the baby on her side, one to stroke the baby, and a fourth to keep your nightshirt out of the baby's face.
- A baby's hands sometimes get in the way of successful breast-feeding. This is because he may be used to sucking on his fingers in the womb and he will try to put those in his mouth now instead of your breast. Swaddle the baby in a receiving blanket to keep hands away from his face during a feeding.
- Make sure the baby's nose isn't squashed into your breast. If she can't breathe easily, she can't nurse. Push down on your breast just by the baby's nose to make a little airway for her.
- Some babies are slow nursers. This doesn't mean there is anything wrong with them or that they don't like you, your breasts, or your milk. They just don't know how to get started. You are the teacher. Within a few weeks, the baby will be a pro.
- Don't confuse the baby by trying to push his face toward

your breast. Due to the rooting reflex, he will only turn
toward your hand and away from the breast. Instead, brush
his cheek with your nipple; this will cause him to turn his
head toward your breast.

- Don't offer a bottle or pacifier to a baby who is slow to
nurse. Don't use a nipple shield. This will only make it
harder and harder for you to breast-feed successfully. A
strong nurser, on the other hand, won't be affected by these
things.

- If your baby tends to fall asleep between breasts, try changing the diaper between sides. This activity will wake the
baby up and make her ready to feed again from the other
side. Some people also suggest rubbing the bottom of the
baby's feet or unswaddling the baby so she's not so cozy
and perks up.

- Problems such as sore nipples, breast infections, and babies
who don't gain weight should be handled by your caregiver
or pediatrician. Turn to those experts who are supportive
of breast-feeding. Otherwise, you may be counseled to give
up breast-feeding. (See Chapter 10 for more on sore or
cracked nipples.)

Breast-feeding Positions to Try

Lie down to feed. This is a nice position if you are sore from
stitches and are uncomfortable sitting up. Lie on your side with
a pillow under your head and another between your knees. The
baby should be positioned on his side, facing you. A rolled-up
blanket at the baby's back will help keep him from rolling onto
his back. Nurse the baby on the bottom breast. In this position,
the breast won't keep falling out of his mouth as he sucks and
stops, sucks and stops. Switch sides after ten or fifteen minutes.

Sit up to feed. Use pillows for good back support. Lean forward
a bit so that your breast falls into the baby's mouth. It may also
help to place a pillow in your lap under the baby to get her better
positioned for eating.

Use the "football hold," so named because you hold the baby in the same way a football player runs with the ball. Sit up and hold the baby with one arm so that his face is at your breast and his body and legs are tucked under your arm and off to the side. The baby is not lying across your lap. This position has the added benefit of leaving room in your lap and a free arm for a toddler who may be in need of a cuddle.

The Let-down Reflex: Is the Baby Really Getting Any Milk? Yes!

Because breasts are not made of glass, you cannot see the milk. Be assured that your milk *is* in there and the baby *is* getting your milk. If the baby were not getting anything, she would not be happily sucking away at the breast.

If this is your first baby, your baby will drink the colostrum that your breasts produce the first two or three days. Your milk will come in between days three and four (the milk comes in earlier with subsequent babies). You will notice your breasts begin to swell, get hard and warm. Get the baby to nurse frequently during the first twenty-four hours after the milk is "in" to prevent engorgement (breasts that are too full).

As the baby latches on and begins to suck, you should feel what is known as a let-down reflex. For most women (not all), this is a physical sensation, like a band tightening around the breast or a tingling sensation. There is also an emotional sensation. You may find youself thinking, "It's so good to feed you. I feel better and so do you." If your milk is coming in, you will see the baby working his jaw and swallowing. He may even let go and choke if the milk is coming in too fast. In this case, you'll see the milk squirt out in a stream. You should not be concerned about the let-down reflex; it is best handled by ignoring it.

If the breasts are soft after nursing, it means that the baby emptied them—even if you didn't *see* any milk or experience any symptoms of the let-down reflex. It is best to feed your baby on demand. This works for animals and it works for humans. If you nurse your baby when he's hungry, you will automatically make enough milk. The chief reason some women don't make enough milk is that they try to schedule the feedings, or they resort to supplemental bottles in place of nursing. Breast-feed on demand and you will be able to satisfy and nourish your baby.

You will know if there is a feeding problem because your baby doesn't act full, won't wet six to eight diapers a day, and won't gain any weight. If this is the case, you will need expert help from an experienced breast-feeding specialist. Otherwise, ignore scientific assessments of your breast-feeding skills. Women all over the world have nursed babies since the beginning of time.

Breast Engorgement

On the third or fourth day after birth, you'll probably notice that your breasts are very full and hard. The breasts may be warm to the touch and the skin may look shiny and reddish. Assuming you are breast-feeding, you can relieve engorgement by nursing the baby often—every two to three hours, offering both breasts to the baby at every feeding, and alternating the breast you offer first. Don't always start feedings on the same side. Alternating allows for a more equally balanced emptying of both breasts. Applying warm washcloths to the breasts before a feeding helps ease engorgement because it can increase milk flow. Or try putting your breast into a basin of warm water before you feed the baby. This helps the let-down reflex.

If you are so engorged that the baby can't get hold of the nipple, express some milk before feeding the baby. To hand-express, place four fingers on the bottom of your breast and the thumb on top. Press in toward your chest and then gently squeeze fingers together, to squirt out the milk.

In general, it's a good idea to always wear a supportive, well-fitting nursing bra for maximum comfort.

Rooming-in

If you give birth at home or if you leave the hospital or birth center within twelve hours of delivery, you won't have to worry about rooming-in policies or practices. If you stay in the hospital for a number of days, however, you may have the option of keeping your baby with you or sending the newborn to the nursery to be cared for by nurses. Some hospitals, as explained in Chapter 2, do not allow twenty-four-hour rooming-in. They may take the baby away at night or during visiting hours.

I encourage twenty-four-hour rooming-in, especially for first-time mothers. It's a wonderful way to get close to your baby in a secure setting—after all, nursing help is just down the hall. I don't believe that putting a baby in the nursery helps the mother to "rest." Newborns sleep quite a lot in those first few days, and you can easily get enough sleep alongside your baby. Babies who spend a lot of time in the nursery go home with nervous parents who aren't yet used to the way the baby breathes, sneezes, snorts, and smells. Mothers who want to breast-feed on demand (by far the best method) will prefer twenty-four-hour rooming-in. A baby in the nursery may be given a bottle by a well-meaning nurse or simply allowed to cry because it's not "feeding time" yet. Whether the baby should be given a bottle or left to cry are parenting decisions that should be made by you, not the staff in the nursery. If you have your newborn with you, you will be the judge of when the baby is hungry or needs to be held.

If your hospital is resistant to twenty-four-hour rooming-in and it is important to you, consider checking out earlier than the standard two or three days.

The Perineum After Birth: Relief Is on the Way!

The perineum is always sore after delivery—whether or not you had stitches. Even an intact perineum is going to burn after delivery. The vagina is stretched out from the birth and there may be some swelling or bruising. If you had stitches, you may be especially sore. The pinching and pain get worse about day four, and then get much better each day thereafter.

For the first twenty-four hours, place ice on the perineum to keep swelling down, provide pain relief, and prevent bruising. Sometimes a topical anesthetic is also prescribed. Every time you urinate or have a bowel movement, use a squeeze bottle (available in drugstores) filled with warm water and pour the water over the stitches. Then pat the area dry.

Let air get on the stitches and they will heal faster. Remove your sanitary pad and lie in bed on a disposable diaper or large disposable underpad to let air get to the area. A sitz bath—a small plastic basin that sits atop the toilet—can also provide relief and aid healing. You can get one for use at home after you leave the hospital or birth center. The warmth of the water and the motion increase circulation to the area and promote healing. Some women use topically applied vitamin E oil to help with healing.

Everyone should do the Kegel exercise after childbirth to increase circulation to the perineum (which in turn speeds healing) and improve muscle tone. For now, work up to twenty Kegels a day and hold each one for one minute. This will be difficult (if not impossible) in the first few weeks after birth. You may think the muscle doesn't even exist anymore. Muscle strength will return, however, if you keep at it. *Do these Kegels for the rest of your life* to tone pelvic floor muscles and prevent urinary incontinence.

The stitches that may have been used do not need to be removed (they simply dissolve). Around two weeks after birth, you may see small bits of string come off with your sanitary pad now and then. This is no cause for worry.

Using the Toilet After Birth

Bowel movements can be scary for many women who are convinced that they will just rip open if they go to the bathroom.

Rest assured, I have never seen or heard of anyone ripping stitches during a bowel movement. Furthermore, it won't be as bad as you think it will be. So don't get all tense and worried. Be sure to eat foods that prevent constipation. Whole grains, fruits, vegetables, plus lots of water in your diet, will make that first bowel movement a lot easier.

Urinating can sometimes sting. This is because the urine can irritate the episiotomy site. A squeeze bottle of water, as mentioned earlier, can alleviate the sting.

Bleeding After Birth

After-birth bleeding lasts for three to four weeks. It is called lochia. In the first few hours after birth, bleeding can be heavy. When you move or get up for the first time after delivery, you may have a clot of blood drop out of the vagina; this can range in size from a golf ball to a large apple. This is alarming but it is only blood that has pooled and clotted in your vagina while you were lying down. If this clot is followed by a gush of continual blood and you are bleeding heavily, call for help and lie down and massage the uterus until the bleeding stops or help arrives.

Over the weeks, the amount of lochia diminishes gradually, turning a browner color until it disappears altogether. There may be days when it turns red again. This usually means you're doing too much (like not getting enough sleep) or working harder around the house than you should. The color and amount of the bleeding are your warning signs to slow down. Pay attention to this and adjust your activity level accordingly. It takes a full six weeks for your uterus to return to its nonpregnant size. This change is called involution and describes the descent of the uterus out of the abdomen and back into the pelvis. Breast-feeding hastens involution of the uterus.

After-pains

Women who have had babies before may notice that painful contractions of the uterus continue after birth. These pains are most commonly felt while breast-feeding, which releases the hormone oxytocin and causes the uterus to contract.

To cope with the pains, there are three things to do:

1. Empty your bladder frequently. A full bladder displaces the uterus and can make after-pains worse.
2. If the after-pains are interfering with successful breast-feeding, you might want to try using Tylenol. If that doesn't help, call your practitioner for something stronger.
3. Wait; relief is on the way. These after-pains will subside considerably after twenty-four to forty-eight hours.

Sweating

Much of the weight you are now losing is in the form of water. One of the ways your body rids itself of excess water weight is through perspiration. So you may notice you are perspiring a great deal more than usual. Just try to keep clean and dry and drink plenty of water to prevent dehydration.

Recovery from C-section

If you had a C-section, you can expect a much slower recovery than the woman in the next bed who had the vaginal birth. Your obstetrician will see you each day you are in the hospital. He or she will leave orders on your chart about what type of diet you may have, what type of pain medication you should take, when the IV or catheter may come out, and when and how often you are to get out of bed. If you have any problems or complaints, keep a list so that you can bring them up on these visits to your bedside. In between visits, the nurses can always call the doctor's office for you to get the orders changed.

Although you are under a doctor's care, your midwife will probably make some postpartum visits and/or phone calls to help you handle the emotional recovery from a C-section, as well as give you any tips she can on parenting, breast-feeding, or making your physical recovery easier.

While in the hospital, take the pain medication you are offered, especially those first twenty-four hours. Try to move around while under the influence of the painkillers. Moving is essential for fast healing but is tough to do once the pain medication wears off. To nurse your baby during those early days, lie down on your side. Place the baby next to you on the bed. You don't want to lay the baby across your scar, which you would have to do if you fed him in a traditional sitting-up position. When it's time to switch sides, get someone to help you move the baby. If you have no help, hug the baby to your chest and roll very slowly onto your other side, placing the baby back down gently.

After you leave the hospital and the staples or stitches are removed, you can usually shower and use ordinary soap and water around the scar line. Keep the area clean and dry. It will be tender to the touch and to clothing for a few weeks. You may want to tape a light gauze dressing over the scar if your clothing seems to irritate the area. The scar will feel lumpy on either side of the incision for several months; this will gradually disappear. There is ordinarily no oozing from the incision line. If you notice a bloody or yellow fluid leaking out, notify the physician who performed the C-section, or your midwife. If you experience any increase in the pain, redness, and swelling at the site of the incision, call this to the attention of your doctor also. Some women develop an infection or have a reaction to the suture material. This can all be fixed; don't panic. You will not come apart. But do call and let your doctor know what's happening.

Once you get past the first week with your new baby, you'll be practically an old pro. In the next chapter, you'll find out about all the baby-care issues that can come up in the first six weeks of early parenting.

10

Crybabies and Cuddle Bunnies

There is nothing quite so special as having a new baby in the house. Newborns are a wonder and a delight—at least most of the time! During the first six weeks, you'll be adjusting to life as a new mother and may have many questions and concerns which we hope to answer in this chapter.

Mood Swings

During the early weeks with your new baby, your emotions will run the gamut from elation to tears and back to elation again. Rapid hormonal changes, as your body returns to a nonpregnant state and begins lactation, are partly at the root of your mood swings. Lack of sleep, anxiety over parenting, and physical discomforts (stitches, etc.) can add to this. It will pass as you settle into a routine and relax with your new baby.

Still, emotional swings can be a bigger problem for women than most people realize and, in certain cases, they do demand attention. In situations like this, a midwife can offer women a lot more time, advice, and understanding than a doctor might be prepared to offer. If you feel unhappy and blue, talk things over with your midwife. She can help you to understand why you feel this way and let you know that you are not alone. If you are seriously depressed, your midwife may suggest counseling by a qualified therapist or psychiatrist. Signs of serious depression include difficulty sleeping, loss of appetite, a desire to remain at home and not see anyone, and unusual irritability with other children.

Midwives usually hear a lot about their clients' feelings of depression for one simple reason: we ask about them. We expect some amount of depression to occur, whether mild, moderate, or severe, and it is part of the midwife's postpartum routine to ask a new mother how well she is sleeping and eating, how many times the baby is waking her up at night, whether she's feeling sad, and how she is coping with motherhood. We start covering the possibility of depression with her during prenatal visits, so she is aware that it can happen. Prenatally, we look at the woman's history and ask a lot of questions about other episodes of depression or visits to therapists. We try to find out whether these emotional problems were resolved, and we warn her that she may be more likely to suffer from postpartum depression if she has suffered from depression before. We tell her that we want to hear from her and talk to her after the birth so she doesn't get so low again. Family members and even friends who have been involved during the prenatal visits, labor, and birth trust the midwife enough to call and tell her when the woman is not coping well. Husbands, mothers, and sisters of the new mother feel that they can come in and talk to me. They know that their input is valued by the midwife because of the way in which they've been included in the prenatal care, labor, and delivery.

Because of this interest, it's easier to pick up on depression early and take steps to help the woman cope with her depression before she has sunk so low that she can't get her head off the pillow.

Care of the Umbilical Cord

Keep the cord clean and dry. The diaper should be folded below the cord stump. Clean the cord stump with alcohol on a cotton swab or with an alcohol wipe. If the baby cries, don't think you've hurt him. It doesn't sting; it's just cold. The cord has no nerve endings. Check the cord for any bad odor. Clean it well until the odor is gone.

Newborn Skin

Babies do not always have beautiful skin. They get rashes and blotches and bumps. Some babies between three and seven days of age get a *newborn rash*, which looks like tiny mosquito bites all over. It may spread over the face, trunk, arms, and legs. This will go away all by itself within four to five days. You don't have to do anything special. Some parents report that their babies look like acne victims. The sweat glands are often clogged on the newborn, and this will produce *pimples*, just as it does in the teen years. Washing the baby's face with a little mild soap and rinsing it well is all that's needed. Also, you may notice white dots on the baby's nose and chin. These are called milia and are very similar to pimples. They are caused by clogged sweat glands. They will gradually disappear.

Babies often get *cradle cap* as well. The forehead and eyebrows develop a scaly crust. This is a buildup of old skin that hasn't come off and needs to be removed gently. Try rubbing baby oil into the baby's scalp and gently rubbing the crust with clean fingernails or a fine-tooth comb. You can do this while the baby's nursing so she won't fuss about it. Shampoo the hair daily and use soap and water on the face to wash off the excess. You should expect to be rid of the problem in a week or so.

Dark-skinned babies may have dark areas across the buttocks called Mongolian spots. These will fade over the coming weeks.

Baby Baths

Before the cord falls off, babies should be given sponge baths with soap and water and then dried. After the cord falls off, the baby can be dunked in water and bathed. An easy way to accomplish this is at the kitchen sink. The first time is the hardest. You'll need a nap afterward! But both of you will soon enjoy the process. Put a hand towel in the bottom of the sink so that the drain won't scratch the baby. Get a big towel ready on the counter, along with a diaper and nightie. Put enough water in the sink to cover the baby to the chest so he won't get cold. The temperature should be comfortable for you (ninety-eight degrees for the scientific).

Babies can be slippery when wet but there is a secure way to hold them. Lay the baby's neck and head on your lower arm and encircle the upper arm with your fingers. Now you've got the baby. She won't slip away. And you still have a free hand to soap and rinse. Smile and talk to the baby. This will eventually be fun for you both, even if the baby cries at first.

You can also shampoo the baby's hair with regular or baby shampoo. Rinse hair under the faucet. Have the towel spread out on the counter so you can quickly cover and warm the baby afterward. When you lift the baby out, slide your holding arm under the shoulders and neck. Pass your other hand under the baby's closest leg, and encircle the other thigh with your hand. You've got the baby held securely now and you can move quickly over to the towel. Simple! You don't have to bend over, and the kitchen counter space is perfect for changing. Remember, practice will make perfect. Besides, the baby doesn't know if you're a little clumsy, having no one to compare you with.

Babies don't need to be powdered. They may need some lotion if their skin is dry or cracked. Peeling is normal for the first few weeks, especially for those babies born after their due date.

Little Boys and Little Girls: Genitals and Other Issues

A baby's nipples are sometimes swollen at birth. This temporary swelling can look very odd to parents who wonder if their little boy has breasts. This swelling is a response to the mother's high levels of estrogen and it will go away spontaneously. Don't be alarmed if the breasts even produce tiny drops of milk.

Girls may have swollen labia, also due to the mother's hormones. Some parents are also frightened to note a blood-tinged, mucuslike discharge from a newborn's vagina. This is normal. Her uterus is simply responding to estrogen withdrawal and bleeding a little. It will only be a few drops of blood for a day or two. Little boys may look odd as well, with swollen scrotums. Again, this is due to the mother's hormones; the swelling will subside over the next few weeks. The pediatrician will check to see that both testicles are descended and will also note if there is any ongoing problem with the swelling.

Sometimes in the first few days after birth, you may notice a brownish-pink spotting in your baby's diaper. These are urinary crystals that will disappear as soon as the baby gets more fluids. They are normal in the first few days after delivery.

Hiccups

You can try to stop hiccups or do nothing. Either way, they will go away on their own. The baby doesn't mind them; only the adults watching feel compelled to do something about them.

Spitting Up

Some babies spit up after every feeding, and in between feedings as well. Others never seem to spit up at all. Both kinds of babies are normal. If your baby is gaining weight at a normal rate, you know he is getting enough to eat despite the spitting up. Some babies have projectile vomiting. The milk shoots out of their mouths and can land two or three feet away. This is truly frightening for parents to see. If it happens only once in a while it's nothing to worry about. If your baby projectile-vomits each time she spits up, then the baby may have a problem called pyloric stenosis. (The pyloric valve in the stomach is very constricted and won't allow the stomach to empty, so the baby vomits.) A baby with repeated projectile vomiting should be evaluated by a pediatrician. In severe cases, surgery can be performed to correct the problem so that the baby will be able to eat and gain weight.

Bowel Movements and Diaper Changes

It would have been hard to imagine before you had a baby that so many of your conversations would now include discussions of the color and consistency of bowel movements. But this is an issue most parents take seriously and worry about. It is very normal for breast-fed babies to have yellow, runny bowel movements. This can make for a lot of laundry because somehow it always manages to leak out of the diaper! This is one reason babies in the hospital wear only a diaper and an undershirt. There is a lesson here: get the baby dressed up only for special occasions.

Some babies move their bowels constantly. Others will go three days between movements and still have loose and runny stools. It's also perfectly normal for babies to have gas and to grunt and turn red in the face while soiling their diapers.

When changing little girls, make sure always to wipe from front to back so that you clean any bowel movements away from the urethra and vagina. Begin again with a fresh wipe.

The issue of cloth versus disposable diapers can be argued on many fronts. Cloth diapers are less likely to irritate the baby's skin and are less expensive if you wash them yourself. They also don't harm the environment the way nonbiodegradable disposables do. Disposables are more expensive, but they are also more convenient. Perhaps parents should consider a happy medium: cloth diapers for use at home and disposables for outings.

Crossed Eyes and Red Spots

As babies learn to coordinate their eye muscles, they will sometimes appear to be cross-eyed. Most babies simply outgrow this problem as their coordination improves. If it doesn't get better as the months progress, discuss it with your pediatrician.

Bright red spots on the whites (sclera) of the baby's eyes are quite common after delivery. These are tiny broken blood vessels. It can take a few weeks for the blood to be completely reabsorbed.

Sleeping

Newborns can have a difficult time going to sleep. They inevitably fuss and fume and work themselves up into a full wail within five minutes. Even when they are sound asleep in your arms, they wake up the minute you put them down. Obviously you can't carry them around all the time, so what can you do? Here are some midwife-approved, mother-tested methods of getting that little one to sleep:

1. Plug in a heating pad and put it in the baby's bed to warm it up. Then slide it away before putting the baby down. The sheets feel warm and cozy, not cold, and the baby stays asleep. Remove heating pad.
2. Instead of waiting until the end of a feeding to change a sleepy baby (an action that always brings him back to life), change the baby halfway through a feeding. This not only keeps the baby awake enough to eat a full meal, but also means you don't have to disturb a baby who has dozed off after a feeding.

3. If the baby has fallen asleep on her side, gently lay the baby in the crib in that position; don't try to flip the baby onto her stomach. Roll up a receiving blanket at the baby's back to keep her from turning onto her back.
4. Low background noise sometimes helps baby sleep: the sound of a fan, a record of ocean waves, of a mother's heartbeat, or of very soft music. Use it whenever you want the baby to sleep.
5. Keep the baby wrapped in the same blanket he was in for the feeding. Don't rearrange it. Use another blanket to cover the baby if necessary.
6. Lie down with the baby and nurse in the middle of a large bed. When she falls asleep, you get up and leave the baby there. It's often the only way to get a fussy newborn to sleep alone! You should put some pillows around the edges of the bed to keep her from wiggling off.

The Cranky Hours

It's 5:00 P.M. From now till bedtime, you often hit the cranky hours. The baby cries, fusses, and seems to want to nurse constantly, acting like he hasn't had a thing to eat all day. As I mentioned earlier, this may be due to the fact that, as a fetus, the baby experienced a lot of movement during these hours. The baby may expect the same gentle rocking that was enjoyed back then as you walked home from work and ran errands, made dinner, etc. Try putting the baby in a front carrier and going about your normal household activities. Better yet, ask Dad to wear the front carrier (after all, you've *already* carried this baby for nine months!).

If you also have a toddler or preschoolers, you may notice that between five and eight o'clock they join in the cranky hour with tantrums. This can make your life even more hectic! Everyone wants to relax after a busy day. We all come home to let go— and yet, when the whole family lets go together, the result can be bedlam. The older kids will refuse to eat their dinners, fight about getting into the tub and then fight about getting out, then argue about getting to bed. For Mom and Dad, this means total frustration and exhaustion!

Try to keep your sense of humor. In moments of calm, see if you can't arrange things differently to improve the cranky hour. For example, feed your children first. Prepare a simple favorite dinner around five-thirty (spaghetti, carrot sticks, and milk). For years at my house, family dinners were marred by spilled drinks, pouting kids who didn't like the food, children tipping over or falling off chairs, and at least one baby who was either nursing or crying while I was trying to eat. Then I realized that young children do not need to eat every dinner with the family. Have your own dinner later, after older children are out of the way and your newborn's cranky hours end. Keep it simple—soup and sandwiches or salad with shrimp and French bread. Believe me, this is better than the indigestion you will get by trying to eat with one arm around a nursing baby and the other trying to stab at your food. When you do eat together as a family, try to make it different and interesting for your other children: a backyard picnic one night, on the living room floor in front of the fire another time. Let children occasionally be in charge of the menus—peanut butter and jelly sandwiches and oranges are nutritious for them and easy for you.

If there's no way around holding your newborn during your meal, cut up your meat into bite-size pieces before you put it on the plate. At least this way you'll need only one hand to get the food into your mouth.

If you can, hire a teenager to come in during the cranky hours to play with the children or hold the newborn while you give baths. An extra pair of hands can be a big help.

Crybabies and Cuddle Bunnies

Some babies are fussy screamers and just seem to be born that way. Others are placid and content and they, too, simply seem to have been born that way. Then there are all those babies who fall somewhere in between and have their good days and bad days. Your expectation of how much crying a baby should do also plays a role. I remember visiting a young couple with a three-day-old baby. I had delivered this baby, and she was one of the ones who comes out screaming. This baby had just wailed and fussed for hours after birth. And she was still at it when I saw her three days later. The parents took turns rocking her and carrying her. They seemed to think this was normal for babies and they were perfectly happy. At her two-week office visit, the mother even said what a good baby she had because she stopped crying as soon as you rocked or walked her! The mother's positive perception of her child made the situation less difficult for her.

Most of us, however, start to clench our teeth after a few minutes of listening to a baby cry. Crying sets the nerves on edge and sets parents in motion to do something—*anything*—to make it stop! As parents, you can become hypersensitive to the sound, so that even the first "eh-eh-eh" out of the baby's mouth can make your stomach turn over and your shoulders shoot up to your ears. Babies who cry a lot make their parents feel tense and inadequate.

I am talking here about a baby who has already been fed, changed, burped, rocked, refed, rechanged, and reburped. Why is this baby still crying? There are a lot of theories, ranging from intestinal problems to hypersensitivity. Sometimes the intestinal tract is immature and you can see that the baby seems to be in pain after feedings, drawing up her legs and crying. If the baby is bottle-fed, try changing formulas or switching from cow's milk to soy milk. Breast-feeding mothers can try avoiding dairy products in their diets in case the baby is allergic to cow's milk. Feeding the baby more slowly with many breaks for burping can also help.

If your baby seems to react strongly to stimuli like bright lights, noises, and people, then stick to a quiet routine. Don't rock this baby. Put the baby down to sleep in a quiet, dimly lit room. Keep voices low. On the other hand, there are cranky babies who need constant contact and movement. They respond best to being held, rocked, sung to. They like car rides, swings, cradles. They respond to music or tapes of a mother's heartbeat.

Their real love is human contact—being carried and watching the world from their mother's arms. Most crybabies fall into this category. Try a front carrier so that the baby can be rocked and held close to you while still leaving your hands free.

If you're feeling desperate and inadequate, memorize this: "I did not cause this problem, I just have a baby who cries a lot." Second: "Things will get a lot better in three months." Most babies who are difficult newborns smooth out around three months when they can begin to interact with their environment more effectively. Music and mobiles will begin to entertain them for longer periods. In the meantime, you can try the following.

Pacifiers: Try different shapes and sizes to entice Junior into latching on to one. Coat the nipple with formula or breast milk to get started. Some parents are concerned about the effect of pacifiers on a baby's teeth. If you use a pacifier for only three months and then gradually wean the baby, there won't be any problem with the teeth later on.

Mothers' Groups: Find a mothers' group or parents' group for companionship. You'll hear and see other parenting styles and can try them to see if they work with your baby. These get-togethers are also great places to vent your feelings and find people who understand. You may get some good advice and support in the bargain as well.

Mother's Helpers: Find a friend or relative who is willing to take over for a few hours while you take a break. You'll return feeling a little fresher with a new perspective on the situation.

Look on the Bright Side: The parenting skills you are learning now will be used again and again as you face other tough times from ages two to twenty-two. Your baby may be difficult to parent, but you are becoming more patient, more innovative, and better able to handle adversity along the way.

Sibling Rivalry

Sibling rivalry is always a big issue for parents. What is the best way to minimize bad feelings? First, try to understand your child's reaction to a new baby. Imagine that your husband brought home a new wife one day. She's a lot younger than you are and everyone thinks she's awfully cute. People bring her presents (nothing for you; you're the old wife). Your husband senses your jealousy (he's very sensitive) and says that, even though he has a new wife, he loves you just as much as before. Now you're going to be one big happy family and he's sure you'll love this new wife, too. He wants you to show her how to do things. "Isn't she darling? Don't you like her?" Of course you don't! So obviously it's not unnatural for your older child to feel jealous in a similar situation. Now that you know *why* your older child might feel jealous, here's how to cope:

- Don't make a big deal out of the birth and the new baby. Tell your child a few basics about how the baby grew and was born, but don't talk incessantly about how the baby eats or sleeps. Let your child ask questions if he's interested.
- Agree that a new baby can be inconvenient and not always that much fun.
- Tell your child about his or her birth and how special it was. Take out baby pictures and reinforce the older child's place in the family.
- Buy small presents for the older child, from the baby.
- Ask friends to bring something for the older child when they come to see the baby. You can continue to do this on birthdays.
- Let the older child hold the baby. Sit the child cross-legged in the middle of the bed with a pillow in his or her lap. Wrap the baby in a receiving blanket and put the baby on the pillow. Siblings really are fascinated by a new baby and want to be close. It makes them feel important. Sometimes, though, they use the request to compete with one another:

"Mom, let *me* hold the baby now, not *her*." Holding the baby can also be a way for slightly older children to handle their strong feelings about the baby. They know they can't hit or hurt the baby so they overcompensate by wanting to hold the baby all the time—whether the baby likes it or not. Set time limits on when they can hold the baby. Let children take turns. If they ask too often, set aside certain times for holding the baby: "Next holding time is at four o'clock." This can take a lot of the stress out of the activity for everyone and you can all enjoy the holding times a lot more.

- Plan special trips for the child with Dad, grandparents, or a good friend. Ask them to take him to the zoo, the ice cream parlor, the movies.
- Make sure the child gets out to the park for plenty of exercise and to let off steam. Don't keep him or her cooped up at home with you and the newborn those first few weeks.
- Make sure you tell an older child at least once a day something nice. "You're so clever." "You draw so well." "That's a great idea!" We all like to be appreciated.
- Encourage and applaud any efforts made to care for the baby. "Thanks for the diaper. You're a good helper."
- Give plenty of love and attention. "Come sit on my lap. There's more room now."
- Expect the older one to hit a rough patch about two weeks after delivery. All the extra attention is gone, as well as most of your patience. You'd like the child to wait without complaining, sleep on command, and sit quietly when the baby is fussing. This is too much good behavior to expect!
- Try to arrange for some household help—a friend, relative, or high school student who can hold the newborn while you play with the older children, or who can play with the older ones while you feed the baby.

How to Avoid Parental Fatigue

During the first six weeks, many women feel so good that they overdo and wear themselves out. Below is a list of dos and don'ts to help you avoid exhaustion:

Do feel free to stay in your nightgown for the first week or two. Clothes may not fit well yet. Besides, once you start to dress and look "normal" all your extra help will probably vanish.

Do not plan to do any major household tasks. Right now, you don't have enough time to rearrange a dresser drawer, let alone paint rooms, wallpaper, or carpet anything.

Do eat meals that you froze ahead of time. When friends ask you what you need, say dinners. There is no greater gift than being spared from cooking during those early weeks.

Do not assume there will be time to study, write, or work on career-related activities. Studying for law boards, graduate school exams, or writing a thesis (or anything more complicated than a birth announcement)—all are equally foolhardy to attempt at this time.

Do arrange for help if you can—either family members or a hired mother's helper. Get someone who makes you feel comfortable. Make sure that this person is willing to help you with the household chores: laundry, cleaning, shopping, and cooking. Don't get a baby nurse who only wants to take care of the baby. Otherwise, you will be doing all the hard work while she is having all the fun with the baby! You'll probably have help only for a week or two and after that you'll be on your own. Use this time to *sleep* and eat healthy foods.

Do not invite people to dinner, lunch, or brunch.

Do arrange for paternal time off from work. A father who is able to spend time with his newborn baby will develop a growing sense of confidence in his ability to parent. Dad will get to develop his very own unique relationship with the baby.

Do not go out with other people for long evenings. If you want to go out, keep it simple—a couple of hours at the movies. Better yet, get out of the house and go sit in a secluded garden or quiet library. You need outings that send you home relaxed, not exhausted.

Do sleep when the baby sleeps. Never use the baby's nap time as your work time. Sleeping should be made a priority in your life right now. Unplug the phone, refuse visitors, and sleep!

Do not go shopping for at least two weeks. You will only succeed in making yourself feel frazzled and hassled. After two weeks, when you do go out, try to arrange to leave the baby with someone and go alone. You'll get errands done in half the time.

Do resist all temptations to be a wonder woman in the first six weeks after childbirth. This is *not* a competition. Take it slowly. You have a lifetime to be supermom. The first weeks are a time of slow transition back to your prepregnant state and another transition into motherhood (whether this is your first or fifth). You will feel much stronger and better rested if you set realistic goals for youself and your family during this period.

Sore Nipples

Nipples can get very sore during the first few weeks of breast-feeding. Sometimes they even bleed. Sore nipples hurt even more when the baby starts to nurse. You may wonder why you even decided to breast-feed. As soon as the baby starts to act hungry, you look for ways to postpone the inevitable. Many mothers also worry that it will hurt the baby to nurse at a cracked or bleeding breast. This is not so: swallowing and spitting up a little blood from cracked nipples will not hurt your baby. And as awful as it looks, sore, cracked, and bleeding nipples are curable. Do not stop nursing when you've got this problem or you may add a breast infection to your list of woes. (The milk backs up and bacteria multiply rapidly.) It's a very tough time. But you *will get better.* Try some of the ideas that follow.

When feeding, make sure that the baby gets the nipple far back in his mouth before starting to suck. Don't let the baby suck on the end only, as this can hurt the nipple. When it's time to switch sides, break the strong suction by inserting a finger into the baby's mouth and firmly depressing the jaw. Don't pull the baby away from the nipple while he is still sucking or you will damage your nipple. At each feeding try holding the baby in a different position (see Chapter 9) so he doesn't suck continually on the exact same spot each time. Also, don't let the baby continue to suck on you just for comfort. A baby gets most of what he needs in the first eight minutes of nursing. Stop when you think the baby's done and switch to a pacifier for the added sucking he may crave.

Between feedings, air-dry your nipples. If possible, spend some time topless. Don't use soap or alcohol or anything drying or harsh on the nipples, as it will only make it worse. Don't put plastic breast shields in your nursing bra. They keep moisture from escaping; nipples stay damp and won't heal. Some women use vitamin E oil to help speed healing. It may be worth a try.

Take Tylenol every four hours for pain or ask your care provider for something stronger. Get lots of rest and take vitamin C (1,000 mg) three or four times a day. It also helps to eat a fabulously healthy diet. Good nutrition builds up your resistance to infection and helps you heal faster.

Call La Leche League or a supportive health-care provider to discuss your breast-feeding problems further. You will need lots of good advice and emotional support to get past this painful problem.

Sex After Childbirth

Go see four different obstetricians and you're likely to hear four different answers to the question "When is it okay to have sex after childbirth?" One will say two weeks, another four weeks, the third will say six weeks, and the fourth will say eight weeks. The answer? I always tell women that they can resume intercourse when they feel ready to do so. A few women will try before two weeks. A few will wait longer than six weeks, but the vast majority of women will find a time somewhere in between that feels right to them. Although you may prefer to wait until all stitches have dissolved before having sex, you will not rip your stitches during intercourse. This would hurt too much and you would stop before it reached this point.

Many women have absolutely no desire to have sex during the first weeks after delivery and only gradually over the months do they return to their normal feelings about sex. Exhaustion, tension, and anxiety—all common feelings for new parents—are not likely to arouse passion. Holding a baby all day long and breastfeeding give women enough touching and cuddling contact; often they don't want any more from their partners. You might want to be left *untouched*. As the baby gets less physically demanding and as you relax into your role as mother, sexual interest will return. Talk to your partner about your feelings so he doesn't think the relationship is in trouble.

If you've had an episiotomy or large tear, intercourse will probably hurt at first. Some women still report discomfort as much as six months after an episiotomy. It can be difficult for the doctor or midwife to see just how many stitches you need and how tight is tight enough. It's tough to make the repair perfect (not too loose, not too tight), so women often end up with a complaint on one end of the spectrum or the other. More commonly, the repair can make you feel tighter, and that can mean that intercourse pinches at first. Try lots of lubrication (KY jelly is good). Be patient. Try to relax. Tension will only make the vaginal muscles contract and make penetration that much more difficult. (I know one labor nurse who recommends a magnum of champagne and a tube of KY jelly to all women who have had large tears or episiotomies!)

Postpartum Exercise and Weight Loss

Every woman would love to leave the hospital or birth center wearing her prepregnant clothes. For most of us, this is a totally unrealistic dream. Don't expect to wear your regular clothes for many weeks after delivery. Try oversize tops and knit, elastic-waist skirts. Or wear relaxed clothes like sweatsuits. They're washable, wrinkle-proof, and easy. Two-piece outfits like this also have the added benefit of making nursing much simpler.

To help tone up and whittle down, postpartum exercises are a must. You can begin tightening your abdominal muscles the day after you deliver. Lie flat with knees bent; press the small of your back into the floor; put your chin to your chest and contract your abdominal muscles. Do four repetitions the first day and increase them by two each day until you reach ten. Usually, by two weeks postpartum, you can start taking walks. Walking is convenient, cheap, and you can do it with the baby along in stroller or frontpack. Start slowly and build up to longer walks. Don't try two miles the first day out and then collapse when you get home! You'll only get discouraged. If the exercise you're doing increases your bleeding, cut back; you're doing too much.

Swimming is another good exercise to take up after childbirth, but wait six weeks to be sure that there is no risk of infection.

Conclusion

We hope this book has helped you to see pregnancy and childbirth as normal, natural, and nonthreatening. Your birth should be the miraculous and joyous process it was meant to be. We've tried to answer all your questions, address your concerns, and—perhaps most important—give you faith in the ability of your body to do just what Mother Nature intended it to do. You *can* have a healthy baby without trauma or unnecessary intervention. We hope your pregnancy will be safe and happy, and we wish you a beautiful birthing experience full of comfort, patience, support, and guidance from those around you. Happy parenthood!

Index